Medical Practice Management

Medical Practice Management

Dean C. Kramer, M.D., LL.B.

Clinical Assistant Professor, Department of Medicine, University of Florida College of Medicine; Attending Physician, North Florida Regional Hospital, Gainesville

Little, Brown and Company, Boston

First Edition

Library of Congress Catalog Card No. 82-81959

ISBN 0-316-50322-3

Printed in the United States of America

SEM

To Barbara, Sara, and Brian

Preface

In eight years of medical practice a number of medical students, interns, residents, and fellows have come to me for advice about going into practice. On occasion some of my colleagues have asked my advice about office management. Having started my own office "from scratch" and established a reasonably successful private practice, I feel that the management experiences I gained may prove useful for those who wish to enter private practice. I have also provided information that may be useful for physicians who already have established practices.

Many practice management books have been written by professional business consultants with no first-hand knowledge about day-to-day medical practice situations. As a practicing physician I have written this book with an emphasis on specific private practice situations that occur daily. Examples of such situations include the handling of after-hour telephone calls, dictating discharge summaries, and keeping track of hospitalized patients. I have tried to provide practical solutions to common problems of this sort as well as to other practice situations.

I have also emphasized the legal aspects of medical practice, not only because of my interest in law as an attorney, but also because of the increasing importance that legal matters have assumed in the practice of medicine. Major medical-legal topics are discussed, including terminating a patient's care, obtaining informed consent, filing claims against a bankrupt patient, and submitting claims against the estate of a deceased patient. The discussion of these medical-legal topics should not be considered a comprehensive legal exposition of the topics involved nor a replacement for the advice of an attorney. The topics are presented to make the practitioner aware of both the potential legal ramifications of conducting a medical practice and the need for obtaining frequent and competent legal advice.

Medical Practice Management does not contain the only method for establishing and running a medical practice. It does, however, offer answers to many of the problems frequently encountered by doctors starting out in practice and by many who are now in practice. Some of the recommendations come from my personal experiences and are uniquely mine. Many have been gleaned from other sources. All are presented in the hope that they will make your life easier, your practice more manageable, and your eventual success greater.

I am indebted to that group of medical residents and fellows who sought my advice about how to start and manage their own private practices for the spark that kindled the idea to write this book.

The production of this book would not have been possible without the extra effort contributed by Harriet Buxbaum, Pamela Hall, and Donna Miller, members of my office staff. In addition to handling the usual day-to-day routine of running my busy office practice, they spent many hours researching, typing, retyping and re-retyping the manuscript for this text.

I gratefully appreciate the assistance of Senator Lawton Chiles for his help in supplying reference material related to the federal government.

I owe a special debt of gratitude and love to my children, Sara and Brian, who temporarily suspended their need for a totally attentive father during the writing of this book.

Finally, I owe more to my wife, Barbara, than to anyone else, not only for her many hours of proofreading, copyediting, and revising, but most of all for her guidance, encouragement, and inspiration, which has sustained me throughout my professional life and made this book possible.

D.C.K.

Contents

Appendixes

Medical Practice Management

1. Getting Started: Where and How to Practice

Deciding Where to Locate Your Practice

Frequently, finding a place to practice takes months of research and planning. Your selection of a location depends not only on finding an acceptable practice opportunity but also on finding an acceptable environment in which to raise your family and enjoy your personal life. Geographic location will be one of the first major considerations. Your personal, professional, and economic requirements must then be matched with the community and practice opportunities most closely meeting your needs.

1. The selection of a practice opportunity involves the consideration of multiple factors. These factors might include the following:

   a. Factors to consider in the community's need for a physician

      The number of physicians in the area
      The types of specialists in the area
      The medical resources used by the people in the community
      The economic structure of the community

   b. Factors to consider regarding the desirability of the community from the standpoint of you and your family

      Available community housing
      Available churches
      Other professionals in the community
      Social opportunities
      Recreational facilities
      Distance to the nearest shopping centers
      Opportunities for your spouse to find satisfying and rewarding employment
      Economic considerations including state and local taxes, living costs, and available banking
      Age of the community
      Weather
      Crime rate

   c. Factors to consider regarding the desirability of the community from a professional point of view

Location and availability of office facilities
The availability of hospital and medical facilities such as nursing homes
The number of qualified physicians in the area for consultation
The availability of allied health professionals
The availability of pharmacies
Opportunities available for continuing medical education
Professional fees charged in the area
Professional opportunities for supplemental income, including working in industry and in school health programs, doing insurance examinations, assisting the public health officer or coroner, and serving as city physician

2. There are a great many resources available to help you narrow your selection. Surveys and monographs on health care data may help you select an area where your specialty is least represented and the need for your services is more readily apparent. There are monographs that deal with the distribution of hospitals, hospital beds, group practices, and average fee reimbursements that you may also refer to as an aid in choosing a location in which to practice (see Appendix 1). Resources that may help you find a practice opportunity include

   a. Placement resources and recruitment agencies

      State medical associations (see Appendix 2)
      National medical specialty societies (see Appendix 3)
      State and federal organizations (see Appendix 4)
      Universities and medical schools (see Appendix 5)
      Health maintenance organizations (see Appendix 6)
      Group practices (see Appendix 7)
      Hospital and clinic management companies (see Appendix 8)
      Executive and professional recruiters (see Appendix 9)
      Consultants to organizations for physician recruitment (see Appendix 10)
      Emergency medicine recruiters (see Appendix 11)
      Other organizations (see Appendix 12)

   b. American Medical Association (AMA). The AMA publishes an opportunity placement register that consists of a comprehensive national listing of practice opportunities. The register is updated quarterly and can be obtained by writing to Physicians' Placement Service,

American Medical Association, Post Office Box 10012, Chicago, Illinois 60610 (312-751-6282). You may complete a registration form and submit it to the American Medical Association Physicians' Placement Service. The basic registration fee in 1982 was thirty-five dollars for non-AMA members and twenty-five dollars for AMA members. The registration fee includes insertion of your resumé in four Physicians' Placement Registers. The fee also covers providing your comprehensive resumé to persons on request and preparing and sending the applicant four quarterly opportunity placement registers from which possible practice opportunities may be selected.

c. United States Bureau of Labor Statistics. This agency publishes *The Occupational Outlook Handbook,* which describes employment trends for physicians. A copy may be obtained by calling the Bureau of Labor Statistics (see Appendix 21).
d. Bureau of the Census. Population trends and concentrations of physicians in a particular area of the country may be obtained from the Bureau of the Census, Department of Commerce, Federal Center, Suitland, Maryland 20233 (301-449-1620).
e. Department of Health and Human Services. Information about the availability and the type and scope of health care in a particular area of the country may be obtained from the Department of Health and Human Services, Public Affairs Officer, 200 Independence Avenue, SW, Washington, DC 20201 (202-245-1850).
f. Miscellaneous informational sources and hotlines

Federal Information Centers (a free booklet listing the nearest Federal Information Center may be obtained from the General Services Administration, Washington, DC 20405, or by calling the Washington, DC, Federal Information Center at 202-775-8660)

National Center for Health Statistics
3700 E. West Highway
Hyattsville, MD 20782
301-436-7016

Library of Congress (Inquiries)
10 First St., SE
Washington, DC 20540
202-287-5205

National Library of Medicine
9000 Rockville Pike
Bethesda, MD 20014
301-496-6308

Federal Job Information Center
Office of Personnel Management
1900 E St., NW
Washington, DC 20415
202-632-6156

Small Business Administration
1441 L St., NW
Washington, DC 20416
202-653-6822

Congressional Information Service
Washington, DC 20515
202-225-1772

Federal Deposit Insurance Corporation
Banking Information and Complaints
550 Seventeenth St., NW
Washington, DC 20429
800-424-5488

Ways to Practice (Solo or Otherwise)

Many articles and chapters in books have been written about group versus solo practice. Advantages, disadvantages, and differences among multigroup practices, partnerships, and solo practices have been pointed out. The benefits of the different modes of practice (salaries, time off, fringe benefits) should all be carefully reviewed in your selection of a practice opportunity, but the major determinant in the decision-making process is your own personality.

If you are compulsive, hypercritical, and fiercely independent, your best choice is to practice "solo." If you are willing to share the responsibility for practice decisions, if you are able to adjust to compromises, and if you can work well with multiple personalities, then a partnership or multigroup practice may be best suited for you (see Incorporating

Your Practice, p. 165). An assessment of your personality needs should be one of your first efforts in starting the decision-making process.

If you decide to join a partnership or a group practice of one or more physicians, it is imperative that you become knowledgeable about what questions to ask and information to obtain to negotiate your contract of employment. Never join a medical group without a clear written understanding of all the elements of employment. Figure 1 is a sample checklist of questions that should be addressed in any negotiation for joining another medical practice.

Your Visit to the Community

Prior to establishing your practice in a community you should plan to set up appointments to meet with the following people:

1. Chief of staff of the hospital or hospitals in which you plan to practice. Discuss with the chief of staff the rules and regulations and bylaws with which you must comply in order to become a member of the staff. Have him give you a copy of the bylaws and rules and regulations to read and review. Specifically inquire about practice privileges in specialty areas, waiting periods before you are allowed to do special procedures (e.g., interpret electrocardiograms), and your commitments to the "service call" schedule in the emergency room.
2. Chairman of your hospital division to further explore issues that the chief of staff is unable to answer and specific questions relating to your area of specialty.
3. Hospital administrator and tour the hospital and the facilities. Inquire whether the hospital is willing to make further commitments regarding the purchase of necessary equipment or hiring hospital personnel to provide for your special needs.
4. A well-established real estate agent to explore the part of town where you would like to live and establish your office.
5. Older established physicians in the community.

FINANCIAL MATTERS

SALARY

[ ] How will my salary be computed?
[ ] Will I have a guaranteed base salary?
[ ] Will I receive additional compensation above my guaranteed salary based on my productivity?
[ ] How will my productivity be gauged; by the dollar amount I generate in patient fees or by the dollars collected by the practice?
[ ] Will I receive a bonus?
[ ] How will my bonus be computed?
[ ] How many years must I work for the group before I reach a time period when my salary is computed by the same formula as other fully participating members of the group?

STOCK OWNERSHIP

[ ] When will I become an owner of corporate stock?
[ ] How much stock may I purchase?
[ ] How will the stock be valued? Book value? Fair market value?
[ ] How much will the stock cost?
[ ] What are the terms of purchase of the stock?
[ ] May I pay for the stock by taking a reduced salary?

GROUP FRINGE BENEFITS

[ ] Will the group pay for all or part of an automobile rental, lease, or purchase?
[ ] Will the group pay for all or part of my malpractice insurance premiums?
[ ] Will the group pay for all or part of my professional society dues, professional journal subscriptions, and professional licenses?
[ ] Will the group pay for all or part of continuing education course fees, travel expenses, meetings, and entertainment?
[ ] Will the group pay for all or part of my office and medical supplies and equipment?
[ ] Will the group pay for all or part of my insurance premiums for life insurance, disability insurance, health and accident insurance?
[ ] If the group only partially pays for fringe benefits, how will the formula be computed to determine the percentage that the group pays?

ACCOUNTS RECEIVABLE

[ ] Will I be required to buy part of the accounts receivable?
[ ] How will the value of the accounts receivable be established?
[ ] What are the terms of paying for the accounts receivable?

Figure 1. Sample checklist of questions that should be addressed when entering into negotiations to join another medical practice.

[ ] May I pay for the accounts receivable by taking a reduced salary?
[ ] If I leave the group, how will I be compensated for my accounts receivable?

GOODWILL

[ ] Must I pay a fee for goodwill to join the group?

TERMS OF EMPLOYMENT

[ ] What are the reasons that I may terminate employment both with and without prejudice?
[ ] If I terminate employment or die, how may I or my estate recover my investment (stock ownership, accounts receivable, and pension benefits)?
[ ] What access will I have to my patients' medical records if I terminate employment?

RESTRICTIVE COVENANT

[ ] Must I sign a restrictive covenant barring me from entering competitive practice in the immediate community?
[ ] If I sign a restrictive covenant, what distance must I move my practice without violating the restrictive covenant?
[ ] If I sign a restrictive covenant, how long must I refrain from entering a competitive practice without violating the restrictive covenant?

MISCELLANEOUS INCOME

[ ] How will payment of miscellaneous income be distributed?

RETIREMENT PLANS

[ ] What are the terms of the retirement plan(s) (eligibility, vesting, etc.)?
[ ] If I terminate employment or die, how may I or my estate recover contributions to my retirement plan(s), and how much of my contribution will I or my estate recover?

PROFESSIONAL, MANAGEMENT, AND MISCELLANEOUS PRACTICE MATTERS

[ ] How much vacation and time off will I be allowed?
[ ] What are the arrangements for weekend and nighttime coverage?
[ ] How will consultations that are referred to the group without a request for a specific group physician be handled?
[ ] How much must I participate in the management of the group?
[ ] Am I required to attend group, hospital, or medical society meetings?
[ ] Must I obtain board certification in my specialty to remain a group member and, if so, within what period of time after joining the group?

Figure 1. (*Continued*)

Inquire about hospital politics and any "infighting" so that you can avoid these troublesome areas while establishing your practice.

6. The last several new physicians who have opened their practice in your community. These physicians will be able to tell you the most recent pitfalls and difficulties that they have been exposed to during the beginning months of their practices.

Preliminary Communications

Once you have decided on the community or location in which you wish to practice, it is helpful to write to the medical society of that county, asking them to refer you to a specialist whose practice specialty is the same as yours. Ask his advice about the need for another doctor in your specialty. Remember that this person may have a vested interest in the advice he gives you and may be "protecting his own turf." His advice, however, may be quite valuable, and he may serve as a source of referrals for you if he has an overly busy practice.

Write to the hospitals in the area requesting a copy of their medical staff bylaws and an application for staff privileges. Most applications will require some supporting information. Such information may include

1. Several letters of reference from colleagues or professors
2. A letter from the chief of service of your medical school indicating that you have successfully completed a training program
3. A validated certificate of state licensure
4. An indication that you are fully covered for medical malpractice insurance
5. Letters from instructors in your training program indicating that you have expertise in specialty areas to support your requests for special procedures (e.g., interpreting electrocardiograms, vectorcardiograms, echocardiograms, electroencephalograms, performing proctosigmoidoscopy, small bowel biopsy, insertion of central venous pressure lines)

Choosing an Office Site

The trend today is for hospitals to help physicians establish their offices close to the hospital. Hospital administrators recognize that the physicians who have their offices close to the hospital generally find it more convenient to admit their patients to that hospital. If you are going to practice primarily in one hospital, it is sensible to consider locating your office near that hospital. Occasionally the hospital authorities will offer enticements for physicians to settle close to their hospital by selling adjacent land at attractive prices to physicians thinking of building their offices. Hospitals may also offer attractive rental or lease arrangements in adjacent, hospital-owned office buildings. When you visit the hospital administrator or administrators in the city where you are going to practice, inquire about land for sale or rental space. The following should be the major factors in locating your office site:

1. The proximity of your office to the hospital or hospitals in which you will practice
2. The distance of your office from your home
3. Parking facilities adjacent to your office
4. The proximity of your office to other consulting physicians, laboratories, x-ray facilities, paramedical support facilities, surgical appliance shops, and any other important facilities

Hometown Practice

There are both advantages and disadvantages to setting up your practice in your hometown. Since you are already known by friends and relatives, they may form the basis for instant referrals for your new practice. It is frequently easier to obtain loans and purchases of equipment in a community where you are well known. An appointment to the hospital staff may be easier to obtain in your home community. There is also that intangible satisfaction of returning to your own community and making your contribution to it.

Make sure that the positive factors, however, are

not offset by negative factors. For example, individuals in your community have always thought of you as the "kid down the street" rather than their trusted physician. You may also find that family and friends are more critical of you than they would be of an unknown physician coming into the community.

An Office in Your Home

Occasionally you will find an arrangement where living quarters and professional offices are combined. Although this arrangement may represent an opportunity for you to deduct the cost of a portion of the living quarters as a business expense, it is generally not advisable to practice this way. Your home should be your sanctuary away from your work and your patients. Your office atmosphere should be entirely professional and without exposure to your personal living habits or family life. You may find this separation impossible to accomplish if you have combined your living space with your professional quarters.

How Much and Where to Obtain Money to Start Your Practice

Most physicians going into practice do not operate their practice at a profit for the first three to six months after starting to see patients. It usually takes this long for third-party insurance carriers to pay insurance claims and for patient volume to increase to a level generating sufficient cash flow to show a profit. Of course, you may experience a shorter time interval before showing a profit; or, if you settle in an overcrowded urban area with tough professional competition, it may take longer.

The amount of money that you will need for initial expenditures is quite variable. Some of the usual expenses incurred by a physician entering practice include the following:

1. First month's office rent and rent deposit
2. Office supplies
3. Moving expenses
4. Local medical society dues
5. Malpractice insurance coverage (usually the first semiannual premium)

6. Premiums for other insurance coverage
7. Cost of personal and family living expenses
8. Office expenses including salaries for the first three months

Most physicians entering practice need to borrow money unless they have available cash resources. Financial theory dictates that you estimate your income, project your capital requirements, and borrow the difference. Since there is almost no way to accurately estimate your income, theory must give way to practicality, and your initial borrowing requirements will be a "guesstimate" at best. Approach your lending institution with the idea that you want to borrow a certain amount but may need to return within several months to increase your loan if the cash flow from your practice is not sufficient to meet your expenses.

You may obtain a loan from numerous sources. The most common source is a commercial bank. Most banks will usually examine your financial statement, inquire about the collateral you have to secure your loan, check your credit, and make contact with the personal references you have listed on your loan application. If you do not have collateral to back your loan the bank may require someone to cosign your loan. In some communities, the bank may grant you a loan without any collateral—a so-called signature or unsecured loan—if you or your family are already known.

You should apply for a loan at the same bank where you have opened your office checking and savings accounts, as well as your personal accounts and safe deposit box. Let your bank know that you have established these accounts and are a potential long-term customer. At the time that you apply for your loan, bring with you a list of any assets you may have. The list does not have to be formally prepared by your accountant, but should include such things as automobiles that you own including any remaining payments, personal items of jewelry, stocks, bonds, real estate, and other things of value. Once your accountant has a complete inventory of your personal and business assets and liabilities, he can prepare a formal *net worth statement* for you.

Most lending institutions will require some form of statement regarding your assets and liabilities when you apply for a loan. Figure 2 is an example of a simple net worth statement.

If your loan requirements cannot be satisfied by a commercial bank, small loan companies may supplement your needs. These companies may lend up to a statutory limit, which varies from state to state. Interest rates are usually significantly higher than those charged by a commercial bank, since small loan companies specialize primarily in loans that are too risky for commercial banks. If you have a cash value life insurance policy, you may borrow against the cash value as a loan. Insurance companies usually allow you to borrow up to the cash value of your life insurance policy at an interest rate substantially below the interest rate charged by banks and other lending institutions. You should consult your accountant, attorney, and insurance agent, however, before you surrender or terminate any insurance.

Some organizations, such as the National Association of Residents and Interns (NARI), provide start-up loans for physicians going into practice. These loans are given at somewhat higher interest rates than those loans offered by commercial banks and should be applied for only after commercial sources have been exhausted. In 1982 NARI offered start-up loans of up to $20,000 to physicians going into practice. The loan can be applied for as early as three months before entering practice and can be used for the purchase of medical equipment, fixtures, insurance, and other business or personal needs. NARI permits a deferred principal repayment option whereby only the interest payments are required during the first twelve months of the loan. NARI also offers loans to doctors established in practice. Inquiries for loans may be addressed to The National Association of Residents and Interns, 292 Madison Avenue, New York, New York 10164 (800-221-2168).

Many of the manufacturers that supply products required in your office offer short-term financing or lease-purchase arrangements (see Leasing or Buying Equipment, p. 48). Leasing equipment or enter-

Total assets	______
Total liabilities	______
Net worth (assets minus liabilities)	______
ASSETS	
CASH AND CASH EQUIVALENTS	DOLLAR AMOUNT
Cash	______
Checking account	______
Savings account	______
Life insurance cash value	______
Savings bonds	______
Money owed to you	______
REAL ESTATE	ESTIMATED CURRENT MARKET VALUE
Homes	______
Other property	______
INVESTMENTS	DOLLAR AMOUNT
Stocks	______
Bonds	______
Government securities	______
Mutual funds	______
Money market funds	______
Retirement savings	______
Other investments	______
PERSONAL PROPERTY	ESTIMATED CURRENT MARKET VALUE
Household goods	______
Automobiles	______
Boats	______
Jewelry	______
Works of art	______
Clothing	______
Furs	______
Other	______
LIABILITIES	
CURRENT DEBTS	DOLLAR AMOUNT
Current charge account balances	______
Rents	______
Taxes	______
Credit card accounts	______
Utilities	______
LOANS OUTSTANDING	DOLLAR AMOUNT
Mortgages	______
Automobile	______
Personal	______
Life Insurance	______
Other	______

Figure 2. Simple net worth statement.

ing a lease-purchase agreement may reduce your need for a larger loan than might have been required if you had decided to purchase your equipment outright.

Ownership Versus Rental of Office Space

A general rule for your first year in practice is to rent an office. Your office needs are unknown, and your financial resources may be limited. At the end of the first year you will have decided whether you wish to remain in the community. There are many complex variables involved in the analysis of renting versus owning an office. These variables include such things as your income tax status, monthly rental fees, mortgage interest rates, closing costs, utility costs, maintenance and repair costs, mortgage payments, property taxes, insurance costs, and rate of inflation. When the time comes to make the decision whether to own your office or to rent, there are several questions that you have to ask yourself.

1. Will the ownership of an office represent a profitable, long-term, investment? Experience says yes. Inflation has kept values in real estate rising over the years, and these values will likely continue to rise in the future. There are also depreciation benefits involved in the ownership of your own office space. Your accountant can advise you about them.
2. Do you have the time, interest, energy, and finances to develop office space of your own? In recent years the building of an office and financing of construction has been made easier by reputable medical office planners and building corporations. These companies assign a building consultant and architect to work with you and provide a "turnkey" job. The offices are constructed and made ready for practice from carpets to landscaping with a minimum of supervision or effort by the investor (see Appendix 13).

Rental of Office Space

The following suggestions may help you if you decide to rent or lease an office.

1. Inspect the premises before signing a lease.

   a. Look for poor plumbing (leaky faucets, broken toilets).
   b. Inquire about the adequacy of heating, hot water, and air conditioning.
   c. Look for falling plaster or peeling paint.
   d. Look for signs of a leaking roof or broken windows.
   e. Make sure that all hallways are well lighted.
   f. Make sure that all doors lock.
   g. Check for the presence of fire escapes.
   h. Have a pest control firm inspect for roaches and rodents.

2. Make a list of damages. Have the landlord attach a copy of the damages to your lease. The list will assist you legally in settling claims for any damages when you are ready to move out and wish to have your damage or security deposit returned. Find out what kind of repairs you will be responsible for and which repairs are to be paid for by your landlord. Make sure these responsibilities are clearly set forth in your lease.

3. Find out if the landlord or management agent has a procedure for dealing with maintenance problems.

   a. Whom do you contact for problems that require immediate attention?
   b. Must you deliver complaints in writing, and if so, to whom?

4. Carefully read your lease before signing. Almost all leases contain formal details such as

   a. A description of the property
   b. The duration of the lease
   c. The name of the landlord and tenant
   d. The due date for the rent
   e. The amount of rent and any late charges associated with late payments
   f. The responsibility for maintenance of the office
   g. The requirements of notice when terminating a lease
   h. The landlord's rules and regulations
   i. The tenant's rights and responsibilities

5. Pay special attention to the following items in your lease:
   a. Provisions for subletting
   b. Allowances for utilities in the lease
6. Remove any unlawful clauses from your lease. Although unlawful clauses in a lease may not be binding, you may be forced to go to court to pursue your rights. It is therefore a better practice to strike illegal clauses from your lease before signing. A landlord who offers a lease containing illegal clauses and who refuses to strike them from the lease when asked to do so may not be the type of landlord from whom you wish to rent. The following are examples of clauses forbidden by law:
   a. A provision that forces you to agree to accept the blame in any future dispute with your landlord, usually stipulating that you pay your landlord's legal fees in any court action taken against you
   b. A provision permitting a landlord to exert unfair leverage on you, such as requesting and failing to return security deposits or prepaid rent under false pretenses or on the basis of unproven evidence
   c. A provision permitting the landlord to assume possession of your personal property for lack of payment of rent
   d. A provision freeing the landlord from responsibility for negligence in case you or your patients are injured on the premises
   e. A provision permitting retaliation against you by eviction, shutting off water, padlocking doors, and turning off heat for such things as complaints to proper authorities about building code violations, and making "do it yourself" repairs
   f. A provision permitting the landlord to force you to continue to pay rent for a dwelling gutted by a fire, tornado, or other disaster
7. Pay special attention to portions of your lease that deal with deposits. When you sign a lease

you are likely to be asked for a deposit of a specified number of dollars—usually an amount equal to one or two months of rent paid in advance. Find out the exact amount of the deposit you are making and the exact purpose for which the deposit will be used. You will also want to know the conditions affecting the refund of the deposit. Here are some things to look for.

a. *Cleaning deposit.* The cleaning deposit is a separate deposit that the landlord is allowed to use to clean or paint the office after you move. In a large number of cases, the landlord does not refund the deposit.
b. *Damage deposit.* The damage deposit must be returned when you leave the premises unless you, the renter, cause physical damage beyond normal wear and tear or cause economic damage by failing to give adequate written notice about moving.
c. *Security deposit.* The security deposit is sometimes used interchangeably with a damage deposit; however, some additional considerations may appear under a security deposit clause. For example, you may be required to rent the dwelling unit for a specified period of time before the deposit will be refunded. Read your lease carefully to see if it contains any provisions, reservations, or conditions affecting refunds of deposits.

Local laws often regulate how a deposit is held by the landlord and how it is refunded to the tenant. These laws may cover items such as interest on the deposit, amount of time before the landlord must return the deposit, and pecuniary damages to be awarded to the tenant for improper withholding of the deposit.

Prospective renters may obtain a free booklet entitled *Wise Rental Practices* from the United States Department of Housing and Urban Development, Public Affairs Officer, 451 Seventh Street, SW, Washington, D.C. 20410 (202-755-6980).

Making Your Move

Whether you are a physician moving to your first practice location or an established physician relocating your practice, you should consider the following:

1. Keep an accurate record of all of your expenses incurred in making your move. Your moving expenses are deductible from your income tax. These deductions include such things as

   a. The cost of transporting your goods
   b. Your living expenses for temporary quarters up to thirty days
   c. Your expenses associated with the sale or lease of your present residence

   In order for you to take advantage of these deductions, however, your move must be in excess of thirty-five miles above your present commuting distance to work. For example, if you presently commute five miles to work, you must move a distance of forty miles for your expenses to qualify as a tax deductible item. There are other specific regulations in the Internal Revenue Code (United States Code Annotated, Title 26, sec. 217) regarding dollar limitations, automobile travel expenses, and other related items. You will want to consult your accountant when it comes time to claim expenses as tax deductions.

2. If you are using a commercial moving company to make your move, select one with a good reputation in your community. Local consumer assistance offices, the Better Business Bureau, and neighbors who have used the services of the moving company should serve as your first line of inquiry. Your state public utility commission, public service commission, or state corporate commission can also provide consumer guidelines. If your goods are being transported across state lines, the move comes under the jurisdiction of the Interstate Commerce Commission (ICC). The carrier must adhere to ICC regulations, which designate the obligations of the carrier and the responsibilities of the shipper. Information about these regulations may be obtained by writing the

Interstate Commerce Commission, Consumer Information Division, Twelfth and Constitution Avenue, NW, Washington, D.C. 20423 (202-275-0854), or from any of the ICC field offices. The following consumer advisory bulletins are available from the ICC without charge:

a. *Householders' Guide to Accurate Weights.* This advisory gives tips on preventing inaccurate weight charges on your shipment.
b. *Arranging Transportation for Small Shipments.* This publication is useful if you decide to ship part of your goods rather than have them transported by a moving company.
c. *People on the Move.* This booklet contains general guidance and a form that you can use to advise the ICC of comments concerning your move.
d. *Lost or Damaged Household Goods.* This bulletin discusses methods for preventing, correcting, and resolving shipment problems.

3. Obtain a free written estimate from your mover. Remember, however, that the charge for interstate moves will be based on the actual weight of the goods and distance traveled according to a schedule of fees on file with the ICC. The written estimate may have an effect on the amount of cash you will need to have on hand for delivery of your goods.
4. Make sure that you have adequate insurance coverage for the fair market value of lost or damaged goods. An interstate carrier has a limited liability specified by law as to the rate he must pay for lost or damaged goods. Movers are not liable for the full value of lost or damaged goods. You should obtain additional household goods insurance if you wish higher recovery limits than those provided by law.
5. When the time comes to move, do not keep old, out-of-date medical books that you have not used for years. Try to sell those books that you no longer use to a medical book store or donate them to a medical library. For those books that you plan to keep, consider mailing them at the postal book rate. The post office requires that

books mailed at this rate be securely packaged in a box, the total dimensions of which do not exceed seventy-two inches, length plus circumferential girth. The cost involved in mailing your books will be less than the cost of shipping them through a moving company.

6. Obtain the following from the driver that transports your goods:
    a. The driver's name
    b. The address of the home office of the moving company
    c. The telephone number of the carrier
    d. The vehicle license number and equipment number
    e. The location of the scales to be used to weigh your shipment
    f. The route to be taken by the driver to your destination
    g. The expected arrival time of your goods
    h. The points where the driver can be reached en route
    i. A final inventory of all your goods and their condition
    j. A bill of lading, which represents your receipt and contract of carriage
    k. The weight of the vehicle before your goods were loaded (tare weight)
7. Plan to be at the destination site at the agreed delivery time. The movers are required to wait only a few hours for you to accept the goods, and less if the move is under 200 miles. If you are not at the destination to accept your goods, the goods may be placed in storage at your expense. The carrier may not, however, show up for an early delivery without your consent.
8. On delivery and *before* signing the delivery receipt, check every article against the inventory to make sure it was delivered. Examine the goods for damage and make a specific written note about any loss or damage on the inventory or delivery receipt.
9. If you have complaints or questions related to an interstate move, contact the local ICC office. For complaints or questions related to an intrastate

move, contact your public service commission, public utility commission, or local Better Business Bureau.

Required Numbers and Licenses

In order to practice medicine and to collect professional fees you must have the following licenses and numbers:

1. *Drug enforcement administration number* (narcotics license). Every physician who administers, prescribes, or dispenses drugs that are considered controlled substances by the Department of Justice must register with the Department of Justice, Drug Enforcement Administration (DEA). A physician who wishes to register must apply for form DEA-224. Applications may be obtained from the Department of Justice, Drug Enforcement Administration, Registration Section, Post Office Box 28083, Central Station, Washington, D.C. 20005 (202-633-1249). The registration must be renewed on an annual basis and prominently displayed in your office. After initial registration, a physician will receive a renewal application sixty days before the expiration of his current registration. In 1982 the registration fee was five dollars per year.
2. *State medical licensure*. You should write to the state Board of Medical Examiners for an application for your state license (see Appendix 14). At this time you should request a copy of the state medical practice act and inquire if a state narcotic license is needed. You may be required to pass a state medical board examination. Many states now have a reciprocity arrangement and accept passage of all three parts of the National Board of Medical Examiners (NBME) testing as a substitute for passing state medical board examinations. There are two basic ways to meet examination requirements for state licensure.

   a. If you pass all three parts of the NBME testing, you will be certified as a diplomate of the National Board of Medical Examiners. Most states will accept certification by the NBME for state licensure. Louisiana and Texas do not accept NBME certification obtained after January 1, 1978. Some states require some other form of reexamination if the NBME certification was obtained more than a certain number of years prior to application. In Arizona this period is fifteen years, in California it is five years, and in Florida it is ten years. Illinois requires reexamination if NBME certification was acquired prior to 1964. The following steps should be taken to obtain a medical license by endorsement of National Board certification:

(1) Write to the medical board of the state in which you wish to obtain a license. Indicate that you are a diplomate of the NBME and wish to obtain licensure by endorsement of National Board certification. The state medical board will send you the necessary forms to apply for a license in that state and a National Board endorsement request card.

(2) Complete the "Request for Endorsement of National Board Certification" card and mail it to the National Board of Medical Examiners, 3930 Chestnut Street, Philadelphia, Pennsylvania 19104. Mail the card well in advance of the state board deadline for acceptance of your application. The NBME will mail to you or to the specified state medical board an "Endorsement of Certification," which the state board will accept in lieu of completing any section on their forms. The endorsement certification provides a facsimile of your diplomate certificate and the scores you obtained on each part of the National Board examination. The first National Board endorsement is free. In 1982 the National Board charged fifteen dollars for each subsequent endorsement.

(3) Return the completed application to the state medical board.

b. The Federation of State Medical Boards of the United States prepares the Federation Licensing Examination (FLEX exam) as a qualifying examination for state licensure. The examination is administered by the state medical board and admission to the examination depends on the statutory requirements of the individual states. The FLEX examination is a three-part test given over three days. The first part is an examination covering the basic sciences. The second part covers the clinical sciences, and the third part tests clinical competence. There are several refresher courses and correspondence services available to help physicians pass the FLEX examination as well as the examination administered by the Educational Commission for Foreign Medical Graduates (ECFMG) (see Appendix 35). Most states require that an applicant for state licensure submit the following types of documents with his or her application:

(1) Proof of completion of an approved internship or residency training program, such as a copy of a completion certificate or a letter from the supervising officer of the hospital where the internship or residency training was taken
(2) Certificate of proficiency from the ECFMG if the applicant is a foreign medical graduate
(3) A photostat copy of separation from military service providing a record of military service and proof of honorable discharge
(4) Two recent head-and-shoulder photographs to be sent with the application (usually three inches by four inches in size)
(5) A letter verifying membership in a county medical society, if applicable
(6) A copy of medical school diploma
(7) Letters of recommendation from several other physicians

Specific requirements differ from state to state and may be obtained from the state boards of medical examiners (see Appendix 14).

You may take the FLEX examination in the state in which you are seeking state licensure or, if you have passed the FLEX examination in another state, you may have the test scores sent from the Federation of State Medical Boards of the United States, 2626 B West Freeway, Fort Worth, Texas 76102 (817-335-1141), to the State Board of Medical Licensure requesting the test results of your FLEX examination as part of your state application.

All states and the District of Columbia participate in the FLEX program. Certain states further limit the use of a previously taken FLEX examination if the examination has not been taken within a specified time period before the state licensure application is made. For example, the state of Florida requires that an applicant resit a new FLEX examination or become recertified by the NBME if the request for state licensure is made on the basis of a FLEX examination passed more than ten years before the application.

3. *Medicare provider number.* You should contact the agency in the state in which you plan to practice that administers the physician portion of the Medicare program (Medicare Part B). This agency will issue your Medicare provider number. The first time your office or a patient sends in a Medicare claim form on which no provider number is indicated for collection or reimbursement of fees, the Medicare office will automatically contact you and assign you a number. There is often a delay, however, and it is best to anticipate your need for a Medicare provider number and apply for it before filing your claims (see Appendix 15).
4. *Blue Shield provider number.* Contact the Blue Shield office in your region to obtain your Blue Shield provider number (see Appendix 16).
5. *Medicaid provider number.* Contact the state agency that administers the Medicaid program to obtain your Medicaid provider number (see Appendix 17). Once you have applied for a Medicaid provider number, most state programs will send you a book of billing guidelines for the Medicaid program.
6. *Employer identification number.* The Internal

Revenue Service (IRS) requires that you file for an employer identification number if you pay wages to one or more employees. Sole proprietorships, corporations, and partnerships must all have an employer identification number. You must file for an employer identification number on or before the seventh day following the day you begin paying wages to your employees (see Appendix 27).

If you call the IRS, you should indicate to the operator that you need an employer identification number for a physician entering practice. The IRS will mail you an SS-4 form. Once they have received the completed form they will assign you an employer identification number. It is advisable to have this number printed on all of the billing forms that your office aide might be required to attach to any insurance claim form. Without this number printed on your billing forms, insurance carriers may delay payment of your professional fees until they receive your employer identification number.

Insurance companies are required by law to provide the IRS with a compilation of all insurance reimbursements paid to physicians throughout the year. The employer identification number assists the IRS in cross-checking and auditing these payments.

7. *Occupational license.* Some communities require physicians to purchase an occupational business license. Telephone your community tax collector to find out if an occupational license is required.
8. *Telephone listing.* As soon as you have decided on the community in which you wish to practice, contact the local telephone company to apply for a listing in the telephone directory. The business representative of the telephone company will inform you about customary listings used by physicians in your area. Your local medical society can also provide you with guidelines for your telephone directory listing.

   Most physicians list their name and office address in the yellow pages of the telephone directory under the section "Physicians & Surgeons–M.D." In larger metropolitan areas the telephone directory yellow pages may have a separate listing for subspecialists known as a *specialty guide.* The specialty guide might include the following sections:

Allergy and immunology
Cardiovascular diseases
Dermatology
Gastroenterology
Hematology

In addition to your name, address, and office telephone number, you may request a listing of additional items, such as

Hours by Appointment Only
Hours: Monday–Friday, 9–12 A.M.
Nights, Sundays, and Holidays call ________
Appointment by Referral Only
Practice Limited to ________

The telephone company will bill you for each line printed in the telephone directory other than your name and address.

New telephone directories are usually issued in January. The publisher of the telephone directory will not usually accept telephone listings for the coming year's directory after November 1. Therefore, if you plan to enter practice in July, for example, you must decide the location of your office and submit your telephone listing at least eight months in advance of opening your office (by November 1 of the previous year) if you want your telephone listing to appear in the telephone directory when you enter practice. Otherwise, your telephone number would not be accessible to the public or your professional colleagues for the first six months of your practice, until the next telephone directory was distributed the following January.

Most doctors in solo practice should have a minimum of two telephone lines coming into their office. The telephone numbers are usually issued by the telephone company in sequence, for example, 732-2468 and 732-2469. You should ask the telephone company to reserve a third line for your possible future use. The telephone company will usually comply with this request free of charge. You should also request so-called rotary lines, so that if one of your lines is busy the call will automatically transfer and ring on the other line.

Some physicians obtain an unlisted private number in addition to their listed office telephone number. A private number permits your colleagues, hospital personnel, family members, and others with access to this unlisted number to reach you without the delay sometimes encountered when calling your listed office telephone number.

Members of the Management Team

The practice of medicine requires numerous ancillary professionals to help run a successful practice.

1. *Accountant.* It is important to have the services of an accountant from the beginning. The major functions of your accountant are as follows:

   a. To set up and monitor your financial record-keeping system
   b. To establish sound financial management guidelines
   c. To analyze the financial growth and trends of your practice
   d. To recommend responsible fiscal policy

   Your accountant will advise you on your record-keeping responsibilities for accurate billing and proper recording of cash received. He will advise you on a disbursement and payroll system to meet the needs of your practice. He will prepare for you financial and management reports such as an income statement and a balance sheet. These reports will show you the financial position of your practice resulting from your billings, collections, and expenses along with the net worth of your practice.

   Your accountant is an expert in tax matters and will advise you on tax strategy to avoid overpayment of taxes. He will prepare the various tax reports you will require on a monthly, quarterly, and annual basis (e.g., your payroll taxes, personal income taxes, and professional corporation taxes). Your accountant will assist you, along with your attorney, in establishing a retirement plan most advantageous to your financial position and needs. He will also file the necessary forms required by the government for your retirement plans. Your accountant will serve as your financial advisor for your investments, particularly as they relate to your overall financial tax strategy and estate planning. Finally, your accountant will represent you if you are the subject of an IRS audit.

Selecting your accountant is like selecting any other professional. Part of the selection process is based on such subjective factors as the accountant's reputation and personality. You can research the accountant's training, experience, and certification. Since accounting is a licensed profession, there are state licensure examinations for certified public accountants (CPA). Acquiring certification as a CPA indicates a certain basic level of competence, but it does not guarantee that the accountant will do a good job. An accountant's reputation can be checked by consulting other physicians who use the accountant or by asking your attorney, banker, or management consultant or businessmen in the community for their opinion about the accountant's skills.

The most subjective factor in the selection process is your assessment of the accountant's personality. This can only be established after meeting with the accountant and judging whether you feel the two of you can establish a good working relationship.

2. *Insurance agent.* When you begin practice, you will need both personal and professional insurance (see Buying Insurance, p. 147). Your insurance needs will require the attention of a knowledgeable insurance agent. Insurance agents may be licensed as certified life underwriters (CLU). Acquiring this certification indicates a certain basic level of competence. A CLU has achieved a certain expertise in the field of insurance equivalent to being board certified in the field of medicine.

3. *Banker.* In the early days of your practice, it will be necessary to establish a line of credit with a bank to pay for your initial capital expenditures. Two bank accounts should be opened: a business checking account and a personal checking account. All business-related expenditures should be paid out of the business checking account, and your household or personal expenditures should be paid out of your personal checking account. These two accounts should be kept separate.
4. *Attorney at law.* Numerous legal documents will cross your desk during the first months and years of professional practice. These include lease agreements, retirement plans, wills, estates, and trust agreements. It is important to select an attorney early in your practice and have all transactions reviewed that may have any potential legal implications. The same principles that apply in selecting your accountant should apply in the selection of your attorney. An attorney's training and certification can be checked in *Martindale-Hubbell's Directory of Attorneys* (Martindale-Hubbell, 1 Prospect Street, Post Office Box 1001, Summit, New Jersey 07901 [201-273-6060]).
5. *Stockbroker.* Although you may not anticipate active trading in any of the major stock markets, several of the brokerage firms offer other services such as the sale of money market funds, the sale of treasury bills and notes, and the sale of federally guaranteed certificates of deposit.
6. *Professional business consultants.* There are firms that specialize in assisting professionals in the management of their offices. A number of years ago these individuals had little special training, but having a background in financial matters and an interest in business affairs, they helped professionals in medicine and dentistry to organize their offices. In more recent years professional managers have established a professional guild requiring that new members have basic training and continuing courses in professional management education to be classified as certified professional business consultants. You may write or call the Institute of Certified Profes-

sional Business Consultants, 221 North LaSalle Street, Chicago, Illinois 60601 (312-346-1600) for the name and address of a certified public business consultant in your area. Management consultants can offer a broad spectrum of services. These services might include the following:

a. Personnel administration including wage and salary payments, performance evaluations, search for new employees, and staff training
b. Analysis of office scheduling, work efficiency, and equipment purchases
c. Establishing professional fees and assisting in selection of office location and development
d. Assisting with accounting systems, budgeting, and cost control

7. *Answering service.* Your answering service will receive calls and take messages during nonworking hours and vacations. The telephone book yellow pages list advertisements for answering services. Some medical societies provide answering services for their members. In small communities, the hospital may operate an answering and paging service for the benefit of the staff doctors. Most services are available 24 hours a day and will answer and screen calls coming into your home as well. The answering service fee will usually be an established monthly charge with additional charges for additional calls above a specified number.

   Depending on your practice, an alternative to the use of an answering service is a telephone answering machine. These machines answer incoming calls, automatically give a prerecorded announcement, and allow the caller to leave a message. The best commercial models of answering machines make it possible for the doctor to call in to his answering machine and screen recorded messages from any other phone location or to rewind the machine and record a new outgoing message from a remote location.

   The costs of telephone answering machines are low compared to the monthly service charge of an operator telephone answering service. The major disadvantage to the use of a telephone answering machine, however, is the loss of human contact provided by an answering service operator. The cost of both an answering machine and a telephone answering service is tax deductible.

Your answering service contract usually does not include your paging receiver, and it may be necessary to purchase, rent, or lease a paging receiver. Paging receivers vary in size from pocket units that are smaller than a package of cigarettes to larger, more cumbersome, walkie-talkie type units that you can attach to your belt. Some of the larger and more expensive units provide two-way communication with your caller. Microcomputerization and rapid advances in the communications field are shrinking both the size of the units and the cost. Smaller, lighter, and more sophisticated communication devices may become more widely available and used in the future.

8. *Computer billing services.* See Collecting Your Professional Fees, p. 187, for a discussion of computer billing services.
9. *Collection agencies.* After multiple attempts have been made to collect your own accounts receivable, it may be necessary to turn some accounts over to a collection agency. Such an agency should be selected with great care (see Collecting Your Professional Fees, p. 187).
10. *Office help services.* There are several companies that advertise part-time secretarial services during periods when your permanent help is sick or on leave. If your community does not have such a service, it may be helpful to contact the personnel office in the hospital where you work to assist you in obtaining part-time help or recruiting full-time personnel.
11. *Notary public.* A notary public is an officer of the state. In establishing your practice you will need to sign numerous legal documents, including wills, lease agreements, bank account applications, and applications for brokerage accounts. These documents may need the seal of a notary public. Likewise, after you have established your practice, and particularly if you use a small

claims court for collection of your professional fees, you will have a continued need for the seal of a notary public. If you must locate and pay for the service of a notary each time it is needed, you should consider having a notary in your office. You may wish to sponsor one employee in a group of physicians within an office complex as the notary public for all.

Applications for a notary public may be filed through the secretary of state in the state where you practice. The requirements for becoming a notary vary from state to state. The notary application fee is a tax deductible business expense; likewise, any fees that you pay to a notary are also deductible.

Notary publics are authorized by law to charge for their services. Most lending institutions, attorney's offices, and hospital insurance departments have one or more notaries among their employees and may grant you the favor of using their services without a fee if you have only an occasional need.

Your Initial Printing Requirements

You will need certain basic items printed when you start your practice. Your various printing needs can be met either by a local printer or by one of several medical printing companies (see Appendix 24). Your initial printing needs might include the following:

1. *Letterheads*. Your standard letterhead stationery should measure 8½ by 11 inches. Your letterhead should be printed on high-quality paper, which in the printing industry means a minimum of 25 percent cotton (rag) content. According to tradition, a physician's letterhead should be white, although there is some attractive professional stationery available in various colors. There are numerous choices of printing styles and types of engraving. Your printer or medical printing company will present these choices to you. For shorter letters, a 7½- by 10½-inch letterhead can be purchased. Both sizes of letter-

head will require matching envelopes. Unprinted second sheets should also be ordered at the same time you order your professional letterhead and envelopes.

2. *Professional cards.* The standard professional card measures $3^1/_2$ by 2 inches. The card can be printed on a medium-weight paper or on a thin light-weight paper. Different type styles and a choice of flat or raised printing are available. The usual information printed on the card includes name, address, phone number, and specialty. Other information, such as office hours and "hours by appointment only," may be added if so desired. You may wish to have the reverse side of your professional card prepared with return appointment information (see Scheduling Your Office Appointments, p. 83).
3. *Statements.* You will need printed statements and envelopes so your office aides can prepare individual typewritten, end-of-the-month statements. You may use regular or window envelopes. You should have all of your envelopes prepared with "address correction requested" printed beneath the return address. For billing convenience and improved collections you should consider a single billing statement that combines the mailing envelope, the statement, and a remittance envelope all in one.

   If you use the pegboard accounting system and your bills are prepared by duplicating the accounts receivable cards on a copy machine, printed statements are not required (see Pegboard Accounting, p. 133). The duplicated accounts receivable statement should be mailed in a "round trip envelope." The round trip envelope provides a combination envelope for sending out the statement that converts into a self-addressed reply envelope for patients to return payments.
4. *An appointment book or log.* There are many types of appointment books. Some of them allow your aide to schedule a whole week of appointments on one page, and others have each day of appointments each on a separate

page. Buy an inexpensive appointment book or log at the beginning of your practice until you feel comfortable with your scheduling routine.

5. *Memo pads.* Memo pads come in sizes ranging from 4 by 5½ inches to 5½ by 8½ inches. It is optional to have these memo pads personalized. The pads are a convenience for jotting down quick notes to patients, friends, and colleagues. Many pharmaceutical companies will offer you free note pads that are usually imprinted with drug advertisements.
6. *Carbon sets.* To duplicate correspondence, your transcriptionist may use either carbon paper or premanufactured disposable carbons with an attached "onion skin" second sheet. As an alternative to using an onion skin second sheet, your transcriptionist may wish to reproduce copies of the original correspondence on your duplicating machine. Although this method of reproduction is slightly more expensive, it does provide a nicer, more durable copy for your records and one that can be duplicated more effectively than onion skin copies.
7. *Telephone record memorandum pads.* There are standard telephone memorandum note pads available for your receptionist to use. These may be ordered from a local office supply company, printer, or medical printing company. After you have been in practice for a while you may wish to custom design your own memorandum pads so your aides can obtain information specific to your practice.
8. *Uniform insurance claim forms.* Medicare, Blue Shield, and most third-party insurance carriers have agreed on a uniform insurance claim form. Uniform health insurance claim forms may be ordered from a medical printing company (see Appendix 24) or from the American Medical Association, 535 North Dearborn Street, Chicago, Illinois 60610 (312-751-6000). Your uniform health insurance claim forms should be printed with your name, address, telephone number, Medicare provider number, Blue Shield provider number, and Social Security number or employer identification number.

PHYSICIAN'S NAME
ADDRESS
TELEPHONE NUMBER

NAME ______
ADDRESS ______
DATE ______

RX	MG.	NO. or CC.	SIG	REFILL & RX NO.
1.				
2.				
3.				
4.				
5.				

☐ NUMBER OF MEDICATIONS

Label All Medications

Substitution Allowed ______

Prior Approval Required ______

PHYSICIAN'S NAME
D.E.A. NUMBER

Figure 3. *Multiform prescription blank.*

9. *Prescription blanks.* A multiform prescription blank is a convenience for most doctors who prescribe drugs. The multiform blank allows you to list up to five prescription drugs on one blank. The prescription blank should have an area for you to designate the number of drugs prescribed. This prevents a patient from adding drugs to the prescription blank. Your prescription should indicate the number of refills that you authorize. You should also preprint on the prescription blank instructions to the pharmacist to label all prescriptions and make drug substitutions, if you agree with this policy. Your DEA number should appear on all your prescription blanks (Fig. 3).

   Prescription blanks can be printed with sequential numbering or in duplicate with "no carbon required" backing to establish a security monitoring system for your prescriptions.
10. *History and registration forms* are discussed on page 89, Preparing a Medical History Form.
11. *Receipt book.* Frequently patients will ask for a receipt on payment of their professional fees. If your office uses the pegboard system, the charge slip also serves as a receipt. An inexpen-

sive receipt book can be purchased for giving receipts to patients who request additional proof of payment.

12. *Office policy booklet.* See Telephone Reception by Your Office Aide, page 86, for a discussion of office policy booklets.

Sending Out Announcements

Pharmaceutical companies may print your announcement as a courtesy. The Eli Lilly Company has been one of the pharmaceutical companies offering this service. You should contact your Eli Lilly pharmaceutical representative well in advance of going into practice to have your announcement cards printed. A week or so before you are ready to accept patients, the announcement cards should be mailed to all physicians in your community as well as to family, friends, and associates. You may use the local medical society directory or the telephone directory as your basic list for doctors and dentists. It is also a good idea to send an announcement to most pharmacists if you are in a relatively small community. If you anticipate receiving referrals from nearby communities, you should obtain a directory of physicians from the state medical society and send your announcements to them.

Advertising the Opening of Your Practice

The American Medical Association Committee on Medical Ethics approves of the practice of putting your name, type of practice, location of your practice, and your office hours in a medical directory or telephone book for purposes of enabling people to make informed choices. A physician may also give a biographical sketch or other relevant data for listing in reference books such as the *Directory of Medical Specialists* published by Marquis Who's Who, 200 East Ohio Street, Chicago, Illinois 60611 (312-787-2008).

Depending on the custom in your community, a brief announcement that you are opening a practice can be published in the newspaper. Your local medical society can inform you about the local practice concerning newspaper announcements.

Promoting Your Practice

In order to promote your practice you should plan to be highly visible during the initial months of practice. There are numerous ways to become known to doctors and patients in your community.

1. Give talks to the local medical society, nursing groups, and hospital medical staff. These talks should be brief, lasting no more than ten to fifteen minutes, thereby allowing time for your audience to ask questions. The talk should not be a definitive exposition on a technical topic. You should avoid the temptation to present a lengthy exposition on the latest research in a particular area. The information you present may be of great interest to some members of your audience; however, there will usually be some people present who have little interest in your topic. You should recognize that your goal is not to present everything known about your topic but to allow your audience to learn a little about an interesting subject and about you.
2. Obtain a teaching position in a clinic, nursing school, or medical school.
3. Entertain socially small groups of physicians that appear to represent potential sources of patient referrals.
4. Join local organizations and service groups. These groups might include your church, Chamber of Commerce, Rotary Club, Kiwanis, and Lions Club.
5. Make an effort to visit the older established physicians in the community. Schedule a five- to ten-minute appointment with each doctor's office secretary. Introduce yourself to the physician, indicating that you are new in the community and that you are available for consultations or patient referrals.
6. Participate in committee work at the hospital and in service organizations.
7. Contact the department of health and rehabilitative services or the equivalent agency in your

state that administers the vocational rehabilitation program. You may wish to become a member of the vocational rehabilitation physician panel. These physicians act as consultants. They evaluate vocational rehabilitation clients seeking financial aid from the vocational rehabilitation agency.

8. Call the medical director of a large life insurance company or health and accident insurance company in your area. Indicate that you are a new physician in the community and would be willing to see insurance applicants that require physical examinations. Your hospital personnel department may also require preemployment physical examinations for hospital employees. Contact the personnel director and indicate your willingness to do these examinations if this is of interest to you.
9. Call a colleague who practices in your specialty. Offer to take his rotation on the emergency room "service-call" schedule. Most physicians are willing to give up this responsibility. The majority of patients cared for in the emergency room on service-call will have some form of third-party insurance coverage to compensate you for your professional services. These patients can form the nucleus of a growing practice.

Courtesies that May Promote Your Practice

When you, as a consultant, admit a patient to the hospital, you should ask the ward secretary to notify the referring physician of the patient's admission. (An example of this would be a surgeon admitting a patient to the hospital referred by an internist for a hernia repair.) This "courtesy notification" allows the referring physician to visit the patient on a social basis, to remain informed of the patient's hospital course and condition, and to comment intelligently if the patient's family should inquire.

If you are referring a patient to another physician, it is courteous to send a note of introduction outlining the problem that requires consultative advice. It is also helpful to send a summary of your records or x-ray reports. Providing recent records and summaries may save your patient many dollars and much time having x-ray films, laboratory tests, and other procedures repeated. Be sure you have obtained proper authorization signed by your patient before sending any records to another physician.

If you discharge a patient from the hospital who has been referred to you by another physician, send the referring physician copies of your dictated history and physical examination, operative summaries, and the final discharge summary. It may be days or weeks before records dictated into the hospital dictation system are transcribed and mailed to the referring physician. You should therefore send a brief note from your office to the referring physician indicating that the patient has been discharged from the hospital. Your note should include your final diagnosis, your plan of treatment, and your arrangements for follow-up. In the event of a referred patient's death, you should express your regret regarding the outcome and briefly outline the hospital course, the cause of death, and any autopsy findings that might be available. These letters should be sent promptly and end with a notation that the full hospital discharge summary will follow within several days.

Get into the habit of communicating promptly with your referring physicians regarding their patients. A referring physician frequently becomes dismayed when a patient returns for an office visit after a referral to a consultant, and the referring physician has no knowledge of treatment, diagnosis, or recommended follow-up care. A referring physician who must repeatedly call you for this type of information will consider using other consultants who maintain better communication. *Build your practice with your typewriter.*

When a patient has been sent to you for a consultative opinion, return the patient to his or her referring physician for continuing care when your evaluation is complete. Doctors have been known to be extremely sensitive about a consultant maintaining the continuing care of a patient who was referred only for consultative advice.

Consider sending the patient a copy of the discharge summary when he or she leaves the hospital if the diagnoses and treatment do not cover sensitive

EMPLOYEES

[ ] Assistant
[ ] Employee fidelity bond
[ ] Personnel policy booklet
[ ] Secretary

EQUIPMENT AND SUPPLIES

[ ] Calculator–adding machine
[ ] Copier
[ ] Dictating machine
[ ] Emergency equipment
[ ] File cabinet
[ ] File folders
[ ] Intercom system
[ ] Medical equipment
[ ] Music system (AM–FM)
[ ] Other office equipment
[ ] Sign, front door
[ ] Sign, front office
[ ] Typewriter

FINANCIAL MATTERS

[ ] Bank loan
[ ] Checking account, business
[ ] Checking account, personal
[ ] Lease
[ ] Moving expense record
[ ] Savings account, business
[ ] Savings account, personal
[ ] Tax calendar

INSURANCE

[ ] Automobile
[ ] Health and accident
[ ] Life
[ ] Major medical
[ ] Office contents
[ ] Office liability
[ ] Professional liability
[ ] Workers' compensation

NUMBERS AND LICENSES

[ ] Blue Shield provider number
[ ] Employer identification number, federal
[ ] Medicaid information
[ ] Medicaid provider number
[ ] Medical license, state
[ ] Medicare information
[ ] Medicare provider number
[ ] Narcotics license, federal (DEA number)
[ ] Narcotics license, state
[ ] Telephone listing

OFFICE SUPPLIES

[ ] Answering service
[ ] Appointment book
[ ] Appointment cards
[ ] Blue Shield forms
[ ] Business cards
[ ] Charge slips
[ ] Day sheets
[ ] Dictionary, English
[ ] Dictionary, medical
[ ] Fee schedule
[ ] History forms
[ ] Index (A–Z) for ledger cards
[ ] Index (A–Z) for files (letter size)
[ ] Ledger
[ ] Ledger cards
[ ] Ledger trays
[ ] Letterhead stationery and envelopes
[ ] Medicare forms
[ ] Miscellaneous insurance forms
[ ] Office decoration and furniture
[ ] Office map
[ ] Onion skin paper
[ ] Payroll ledger
[ ] Payroll withholding booklets
[ ] Pegboard system
[ ] Petty cash box (or safe)
[ ] *Physicians' Desk Reference*
[ ] Postal scales
[ ] Prescription pads
[ ] Receipt book
[ ] Relative value studies
[ ] Return envelope combination ("round-trip" envelopes)
[ ] Signs, office informational
[ ] Zip code directory

PROFESSIONAL PROMOTION

[ ] Announcements
[ ] Contacts for referrals
[ ] Hospital privileges
[ ] Medical memberships, county and state
[ ] Memberships, civic and church

Figure 4. Basic checklist for going into practice.

areas. Many patients like to have a copy of their medical records and appreciate your thoughtfulness in sending their records to them. Legally, patients are entitled to a full disclosure of test results and diagnoses, providing the information does not do them more harm than good. If the diagnoses involve sensitive areas such as psychiatric conditions and severe illnesses, you may rely on direct communication at the time the patient leaves the hospital rather than sending the full disclosure in your discharge summary in the mail.

Your best practice builder is the delivery of kind, thoughtful, high-quality professional care. This level of care always results in word-of-mouth recommendations from one patient to another and the growth of a successful practice.

A summary of the basic items you will need to set up your practice is presented in Figure 4.

2. *Office Planning and Development*

Planning Your Office

1. *Office Decor.* Your office decor should project your professional image. Consider hiring the services of an interior designer to assist you in the selection of your office's color scheme; wall, floor, and window coverings; furniture; and accessories. A few basic concepts will help you approach your office planning more efficiently.

   a. Color can influence the illusion of space. Light colors tend to create the feeling of a larger room. Rich earth tones, like orange, brown, and beige, give a feeling of warmth and tranquility.
   b. Office furnishings should be attractive and of high quality construction. Furnishings should be color coordinated with the interior of the room, as well as functional and comfortable.
   c. Floor coverings should be attractive and create a minimum of maintenance problems. A commercial grade of wall-to-wall carpeting is attractive as well as practical. This type of carpeting may be your best choice for reception rooms, hallways, consultation rooms, and possibly your examining rooms if you do not anticipate frequent spillage on the floor. In areas of heavy traffic and anticipated spillage (e.g., the business office, laboratory, and treatment room), linoleum, cork, rubber, asphalt, plastic tile, or permanent terrazzo provide the best choices for floor coverings.

2. *Office areas.* There are certain basic office areas that are common to all physicians' offices. These areas include the following:

   a. *Reception room.* Depending on your type of practice, your reception room or waiting area may occupy a large portion of your office space. There are general guidelines for establishing the seating and space requirements for your reception room. Since patients frequently bring friends and relatives with them to the office, a safe rule of thumb is to provide seating for three times the number of individuals that you have scheduled to see in an hour's time. Office planners usually recommend that your reception room be sixty square feet plus ten square feet of seating space for each person as a minimum guideline for overall room size. For example, if you plan to see four patients in an hour you should plan to have twelve seating spaces in a reception room measuring a minimum of 180 square feet. It is natural for strangers not to wish to sit next to other strangers in a doctor's office. Plan your type of seating accordingly. Avoid couches and concentrate on sturdy, comfortable, and attractive single seating units.

Besides seating, your reception room should include a magazine rack, and, of course, magazines. General interest magazines like *Ladies' Home Journal, Reader's Digest, Time, Life,* and *Good Housekeeping* provide interesting and suitable material for your reception room. There are companies that specialize in providing reception room subscription services. By using such a service you will have the added convenience of making one order, writing one check, and having one renewal time. The services advertise a common expiration date so that all of the subscriptions are renewed at the same time. Several weeks or months before the subscriptions expire the company will usually send a renewal notice. This single renewal notice reduces the need to screen multiple copies of publishers' renewal notices throughout the year. Subscriptions to most popular reception room magazines are usually offered through these services. An example of one reception room subscription service is EBSCO, Reception Room Subscription Service, 5350 Alpha Road, Dallas, Texas 75250 (800-527-5901). EBSCO and other subscription agencies also offer similar subscription services for ordering all of your professional medical journals (see Appendix 37).

Background music from an inexpensive FM receiver can provide a pleasant and relaxing atmosphere for patients who are generally tense in a doctor's reception room. Companies such as Muzak, Division of Teleprompter Corporation, 888 Seventh Avenue, New York, New York 10106 (212-247-3333), specialize in installing sound systems that provide continuous instrumental background music.

Tasteful wall covering, pictures, accessories, plants, and carpeting will add to the overall effect and provide the image that you wish to project. Your reception room should have an area for your patients to hang their coats, hats, and umbrellas. You should also try to provide access in your waiting room to a water fountain and restroom. In order to maintain control and monitor access to the restroom, it should be within view of your front office aides.

A telephone in your reception room is a convenience for the use of your patients. The telephone company can install a telephone line in your reception room that can be used for local calls only.

b. *Consultation room.* Although it is not an absolute requirement that you have a consultation room separate from your examining rooms, it does provide a room for you to carry on your business activities and have private conferences and interviews "away from the traffic." It may also provide an area for you to store your library and hang your diplomas.

c. *Examination rooms.* Examining rooms are necessary for most internists, surgeons, and family practitioners. The minimum practical size for an examination room is ninety-six square feet. A number of time and motion studies suggest that three examining rooms are the ideal number for patient flow for most internists, surgeons, and general practitioners. For these types of physicians, the examination room should include an examining table, sink, a chair for both doctor and patient, a waste receptacle, writing surface, and some form of storage cabinetry. It is a convenience for the patient to have a small area in which to hang clothes and dress in privacy. A simple track stapled into the ceiling in one corner of the room with a curtain designed to pull will provide the required privacy. Consider installing a chart rack outside each examination room near the entry door.

Subspecialists, such as ophthalmologists, otolaryngologists, and psychiatrists will have special size and equipment needs. A separate room in which to perform surgical procedures may be required by physicians in some specialties. The space and equipment needs for these rooms must be custom designed to the needs of each physician.

d. *Business office*. Your business office should at least equal the size of your consultation room. You should always include plans for future expansion and additional office personnel, new equipment, and storage space in the business office. As your practice grows, the need for an expanded business office will grow as well. The business office is the area where future space needs are most often underestimated. You should reserve 100 to 300 square feet of space for future expansion needs. A good rule of thumb is to provide 125 square feet of business office space for one office aide and 75 square feet for each additional aide that works in your business office.

e. *Restrooms*. A restroom for patients and a private restroom for your office aides should be incorporated in your office plans. It is important in new construction to make sure that the restrooms are wide enough to accept a wheelchair for handicapped patients. Most building codes now require this design. If you are building a new office or remodeling an old one, consider making a pass-through space between the wall of the restroom and the laboratory or nursing station. This opening gives the patient the opportunity to leave urine specimens in a location that can be easily reached by your office aide with a minimum of patient handling and embarrassment.

f. *Storage areas.* Planning for storage is one of the most neglected items of consideration during the allocation of space. When you start out in practice, storage will not seem to be a major problem; however, after years of accumulating files and supplies, storage space becomes limited. You should plan to have storage closets and space identified for the future growth of your practice. A separate closet or an area in your office should also be set aside for drug samples (see Pharmaceutical Company Representatives, p. 62). You should plan another storage area for patient information literature. It is from this central file of stored literature that you can stock examination and reception rooms with information handouts.

g. *Laboratory.* Depending on your type of practice, you may either want to do a large number of laboratory procedures in your office or to have your patients go to a nearby laboratory to have their tests performed. Some physicians prefer to draw their patients' blood and send the blood to an out-of-town laboratory for processing.

   If your patients have blood drawn at a local laboratory or if you mail most of your patients' blood samples away for processing, your space needs for laboratory and equipment will be minimal. The simplest office laboratory might contain a microhematocrit centrifuge, a small multipurpose centrifuge, a microscope, and urinalysis testing materials with necessary glassware.

h. *Corridors.* Your office corridors should be wide enough to allow two people to pass each other comfortably. You should allow a minimum width of forty-four inches, but preferably five feet for most of your office corridors.

There are several excellent free guides to assist you with developing your space needs. These guides may be obtained from the American Medical Association, 535 North Dearborn, Chicago, Illinois 60610 (312-751-6000), and the American Surgical Trade Association, 11 East Adam Street, Chicago, Illinois 60603 (312-427-2577).

Leasing or Buying Equipment

You may spend a sizeable amount of money to purchase your initial office equipment. The question often arises whether you should lease, buy, or obtain a loan to purchase your equipment. Your cash flow will determine which of these options is best for you. There is universal agreement that for most physicians starting in practice the least expensive way to obtain equipment is direct purchase. However, a loan or a lease with an option to purchase, although more expensive, requires less cash outlay and may be advantageous during your early years of practice.

If you lease equipment, make sure your lease includes an option to buy the equipment at the end of the lease. Also make sure that the option to purchase for "fair market value" at the end of the lease is not overinflated. For example, the fair market value at the end of a three-year lease of equipment may reasonably be 15 percent of the original purchase price, but not 75 percent.

Try to get a clause in your agreement allowing you to cancel your equipment lease if a newer model that you wish to purchase is introduced, or to include an option to negotiate a new lease for a newer model.

Your lease should specify who is responsible for maintenance, repairs, and casualty losses, as well as who pays the personal property taxes, if any, on the equipment if it is purchased. Always discuss the lease with your accountant and have the lease document reviewed by your attorney.

Buying Office Furniture and Equipment

The hospital where you practice may have an arrangement with a local office supply company for the purchase of furniture and supplies. Check with the administrator of the hospital to find out if you can ethically and legally take advantage of the hospital's purchasing contracts. If the hospital does not have such an arrangement, you may wish to negotiate a discount with a local office supply company for your first large expenditure for furniture and equipment.

Business Office Equipment

There are certain essential pieces of business office equipment that you should purchase.

1. *Typewriter.* Your front office aides will require a typewriter. Typewriters can be purchased for as little as $75 and as much as $1,500 or more depending on your desire for convenience features. You should invest in an electric typewriter to give your correspondence the nicest appearance and your typist the most convenience. A self-correcting feature offered on some electric typewriters is a time-saving extra that will pay for itself. As an example, the IBM Selectric typewriter series represents some of the best units on the market. If you anticipate the need for reproducing forms or letters, there are also typewriters available with computer memory features that will produce your documents automatically. As with all major office equipment purchases, a maintenance contract is advisable. The maintenance contract will usually cost about 10 percent of the actual purchase price per year.
2. *Printing calculator.* An electric printing calculator can be purchased for less than $100. Your office financial secretary should require only the basic functions of addition, subtraction, multiplication, and division. More expensive units can be purchased if additional features are required. It is important that the unit you purchase produce a paper tape, so that you, your accountant, or your management consultant can review calculations. The tape also simplifies finding errors if they occur.
3. *Office copier.* An office copier has become an almost indispensable part of an efficient business office. A copier is needed to duplicate such things

as a patient's records to send to other physicians, records and forms for insurance companies, records and billing information for patients, and a patient's account receivable card for end-of-the-month billing. There are three basic types of copiers:

a. Copiers that use plain paper versus chemically coated paper
b. Copiers that are sheet fed versus roll fed
c. Copiers that have a dry development process versus a wet development process

Copiers may have any number of combined characteristics. For example, plain paper, sheet fed, dry development process; plain paper, sheet fed, wet development process; or chemical coated paper, roll fed, wet development process. There are advantages and disadvantages to each characteristic. Your copier salesman will point these out to you. You should select a copier after reviewing the features of several machines with varying characteristics. Attention should be paid particularly to the quality of the reproduction and the ability of the machine to rapidly reproduce the type of originals that your office most often copies with minimum potential for paper jams and breakdowns. Have your local sales representatives demonstrate the machines to you and your office aides and leave a machine in your office for a trial period.

Some of the major manufacturers of high-quality equipment include Canon, Eastman Kodak, IBM, Minolta, 3M, Pitney Bowes, Savin, Sharp, Royal, and Xerox (see Appendix 29).

As with all front office equipment, the ability to obtain local maintenance service and a "loaner" if your equipment is inoperative are major considerations. You should also purchase a maintenance service contract for your copier. The cost of a high-quality, desk model copier ranged from $1,000 to $3,000 in 1982.

4. *Dictation equipment.* You may require some form of dictation system in your office. There are a number of systems that can be adapted to your personal needs. The simplest system is a desk-

top, dictation-transcription unit. Almost all desktop units manufactured today serve interchangeably as a dictation unit and a transcription unit. If your dictation requirements are minimal when you start practice and if your budget for equipment purchases is limited, you may consider buying a single dictation-transcription unit and having the unit shuttled back and forth between your desk and the desk of your transcriptionist. Eventually you can have separate units for both you and your transcriptionist. The cost of a high-quality dictation-transcription unit ranged from $450 to $650 in 1982.

Some physicians enjoy the flexibility of carrying portable dictation units. These units are small, lightweight, and portable and may be used to dictate both inside and outside the office. Recent advances have miniaturized dictation units to the size of a cigarette case and microcassettes to the size of two postage stamps. Larger portable units are available to use with standard cassettes.

A more elaborate system that adapts well to a multiple physician office is the multiple dictation input system with a central recorder. Multiple dictating stations may be located throughout the office and dictated into from either a microphone-type input or a telephone-type input. The choice of input style is one of personal preference. The person dictating can record, stop, rewind, and correct. A central recorder consisting of a continuous loop of tape receives the dictation and allows the transcriptionist working at one of the stations to type almost simultaneously as you dictate. A continuous loop system cost between $1,200 and $1,500 in 1982, with varying additional charges, depending on the number of input units required. You may wish to pay extra for certain convenient optional features, such as the telephone call-in feature, which allows you to connect your office telephone to the continuous loop recorder. You can then dictate messages from outside your office, thereby recording them for future transcription. A few of the major companies specializing in dictation and transcription equipment include Dictaphone, IBM, Lanier, Norelco, Sony, and Sanyo (see Appendix 19).

5. *Postage meters.* A postage meter is a convenience and a luxury, but not a necessity, in the front office. When you start out in practice, the volume of mail posted will be limited. During the first months of practice the amount paid for monthly rental on a postage meter may exceed your whole month's postage bill. As your practice grows and the volume of your mail increases, you may find it convenient and more economical to have a postage meter, particularly if you find that your office aide must drive several times each month to the post office to buy stamps.

   A postage meter may not be a necessity in your office, but it is important to have a postage scale. An inexpensive scale can be purchased from an office supply company for less than ten dollars. Over the years your postage scale can save you money. Your office aides will be able to add accurate amounts of postage to your mail without overpaying or having the mail returned for postage due. Your scales should be checked for accuracy at intervals. A handful of change is all that is required to check the accuracy of your scales. Each of the following sets of coins weighs one ounce: nine pennies, twelve dimes, or five quarters.
6. *Check protector.* A check protector embosses your checks with the amount, thereby making it difficult or impossible to alter. It is a convenience, but not a necessity, to have a check protector. If you do not use a check protector, when your checks are prepared, you should make a special effort to thumb through your end-of-the-month cancelled checks to make sure no alterations have been made. Do not give this responsibility to your office aides since this is your means to assure yourself that no staff member is responsible for any alterations made on checks.
7. *Telephones.* There are two ways to obtain telephone service in your office. The first is to lease your telephone hardware (e.g., telephones, chimes, intercom) from your local public telephone company or from a private telephone equipment manufacturer. The second way to obtain service is to buy your telephone hardware from your local public telephone company or

from a private telephone equipment manufacturer.

a. *Buying your telephone equipment.* Buying your own telephone system hardware either from your local public telephone company or from a private manufacturer offers several advantages over leasing your telephone equipment. Some of these advantages include
   (1) Equity in your telephone hardware
   (2) Tax depreciation allowances
   (3) Investment tax credits for new business equipment purchases
b. *Leasing your telephone equipment.* If you are a physician starting in practice with limited cash flow, you may wish to lease your telephone system equipment from the company that you select to install your equipment (either the local public telephone company or another telephone communication system manufacturer). Leasing your telephone equipment provides you with the telephone service you need with a minimum outlay of cash. Your lease should provide for the following (see also Leasing or Buying Equipment, p. 48):

   (1) The option to buy the telephone hardware at the termination of the lease at a fair market value
   (2) The option to upgrade the equipment to a more sophisticated system, if required
   (3) A maintenance agreement to handle all repairs and replacements for equipment failures

c. *Optional features.* Aside from the basic telephone equipment, many convenient optional features can be added to your telephone system at additional costs. Some of the optional features include

   (1) Hold key
   (2) Intercom
   (3) Music on "hold"
   (4) Conference call capability
   (5) Computerized speed-dialing
   (6) Call forwarding

You should contact several communication system manufacturers in your area and compare their equipment, optional features, prices, and service contracts with those offered by your local public telephone company. Two of the larger private telephone manufacturing companies are Executone, Two Jericho Plaza, Jericho, New York 11753 (800-243-4311), and International Telephone and Telegraph (ITT), Telecom Drive, Milan, Tennessee 38358 (901-686-7401).

As your practice grows, the volume of telephone calls will invariably increase. If you suspect that many patients are reaching a busy signal when they call your office, you may ask the telephone company to do a "busy signal survey," which they will usually carry out without charge. If more than 20 percent of your patient calls result in a busy signal, you should consider adding new lines to your office system or reevaluating your office aides' handling of telephone calls.

A noteworthy, time-saving piece of telephone equipment that can be ordered from your local telephone company is an automatic dialer or speed-dialer. Your telephone can be programmed to retain from eight to thirty of your most frequently called numbers. With the push of a button a number can be automatically dialed. The programmed number and the names of the callers are displayed on the front panel of the telephone for easy referral (see also Required Numbers and Licenses, Telephone Listing, p. 25). Speed-dialers may also be purchased from private manufacturers like the Tandy Corporation, Post Office Box 1052, Fort Worth, Texas 76102 (817-390-3700), through their retail distribution outlet, Radio Shack. The speed-dialers can be connected to your leased or purchased telephone hardware.

Filing Storage Equipment

There are two kinds of filing storage systems.

1. *Open shelf filing.* This form of filing system consists of a series of horizontal open shelves con-

structed to hold your medical files. Open shelf files are available in various heights and widths. Typical shelf units contain five bins and are at least sixty inches high, ranging from thirty to forty-two inches in width and thirteen to seventeen inches in depth. Some open shelf filing systems come as modular units. These modular units offer greater filing capacity per unit space than a closed filing cabinet. The modular units are easy to assemble and can be expanded as your need for filing space grows. Modular units allow for the potential use of all the floor to ceiling space delegated for filing in your office. The advantages of an open shelf filing system are the following:

a. Time and energy are saved and noise is reduced because it is not necessary to open and close filing drawers.
b. Open shelf files are less expensive to purchase than closed shelf filing cabinets.
c. More charts are exposed at any one time so it is easier for your office aide to find and refile charts quickly.

2. *Closed cabinet filing.* Closed cabinet filing systems come in two styles, lateral files and vertical files. *Lateral filing* cabinets are usually placed against a wall, but may, however, be used as attractive area dividers. The file drawers glide out about a foot toward the filing clerk so aisles can therefore be narrower with the use of lateral files than with vertical files. In a lateral filing system the front of each folder faces the side of the file drawer as opposed to a vertical file system, in which the front of each folder faces the front of the file drawer.

   Vertical files can be purchased in different drawer heights. At the maximum height of five drawers, a vertical file is estimated to hold about seven hundred records. Extra aisle space must be allowed if this type of file drawer is to be fully extended. If you purchase a vertical file, it should have ball bearing, roller suspension for each drawer. Inexpensive file cabinets can be purchased without ball bearing, roller suspension drawers, but they represent a false economy because of the extra effort required to close the file drawers.

The advantages of a closed filing cabinet system include the following:

a. The closed cabinet file can be constructed with a locking device, thereby offering protection against theft and vandalism as well as ensuring confidentiality of patient records within a closed, locked area.
b. The closed cabinet file can be insulated for fire protection.
c. The closed cabinet file protects records from dirt and dust.
d. The closed cabinet file is usually neater and more orderly than an open shelf filing system (see Appendix 20).

Filing Systems

The two basic ways to establish a filing system are the alphabetical filing system and the numerical filing system.

1. *The alphabetical filing system.* In an alphabetical filing system records are filed in order of the alphabetical sequence of letters in the patient's last name. Records stored in this manner can be retrieved directly from the files without reference to the separate index required with a numerical system. The alphabetical filing system is recommended for solo practitioners and small group practices.

   a. The possible disadvantages of an alphabetical filing system include

      (1) Difficulty finding charts owing to misspellings of last names
      (2) Difficulty finding charts owing to clerical errors in alphabetical filing
      (3) Difficulty retrieving records of patients with common last names

   b. The possibility of errors can be reduced in an alphabetical filing system by establishing filing rules to be followed by all of your office aides. Examples of filing rules might include the following:

(1) Type the patient's last name, first name, and middle initial on a gummed label and attach it to the side tab of the file (see also Constructing the Office Chart, p. 94). Avoid handwritten identification labels.
(2) File alphabetically according to surname, given name, and middle initial or name.
(3) Treat compound and hyphenated surnames as one word.
(4) Disregard titles.
(5) File the records of married women according to their legal signature rather than their husband's name.
(6) File the records of patients that use initials for their first name alphabetically before patients with an identical surname that have a full given name; for example, *Thompson, P.* is filed before *Thompson, Paul.*

2. *The numerical filing system.* In a numerical filing system each new patient is given a sequential number. The numerical system requires an alphabetical cross-index to obtain the patient's chart number. The alphabetical cross-index may be prepared as cards mounted on rotating wheels (Rolodex type), on panels, or filed in a drawer or special filing cabinet. It is not advisable to use the patient's account receivable card as the alphabetical cross-index. If an account receivable card is misplaced, your office aide will not be able to find the patient's chart number or chart.

   For those physicians' offices that use a numerical system, the straight sequential numerical system is adequate. There are more complicated numerical systems based on middle and terminal digit filing that are used primarily by large group practices and hospitals. The numerical system has the advantage of reducing the number of misfiled charts and is best adapted for use by hospitals and large group practices with thousands of files.

Color-coding of files has been introduced to reduce filing errors. Errors may be more readily identified through visual recognition of a misfiled chart (see also Constructing the Office Chart, p. 94). Color-coding of files may be used with either the alphabetical or the numerical filing system. Colored files may be assigned to certain groups of alphabetical letters. For example, letters A through D could be color-coded red, letters E through H color-coded blue, and so on. Color-coded filing systems may be purchased from medical printers and office supply companies (see Appendix 24).

The latest advances in filing systems, filing equipment, and other business equipment and systems are featured in the monthly publication *Office Product News*. This publication may be obtained free of charge by writing to Hearst Business Communications, U.T.P. Division, 645 Stewart Avenue, Garden City, New York 11530 (516-222-2500).

Protecting Records and Valuables

If you have not purchased a fire-insulated filing cabinet with a locking device, it is advisable to purchase an insulated safe. In 1982, small floor models could be purchased for less than $200. Safes and fire-insulated filing cabinets can usually be purchased through an office supply company. The companies that specialize in manufacturing home and office safes include Sentry, 900 Lyndon Avenue, Rochester, New York 14625 (716-381-4900), and Morgan Safe Company, 811 Second Avenue, New Hyde Park, New York 11040 (212-658-6774).

Your safe will make an excellent repository for any narcotics that you keep in the office that do not need refrigeration. You should also keep in the office safe your petty cash fund, postage stamps, postage meter, and any valuable documents that may temporarily pass through your office, such as stocks and bonds, prior to transfer to your safe deposit box. The purchase of a safe for your office is a tax deductible expense.

It is particularly important to store your accounts receivable records in a fire-insulated locked cabinet or safe when your office is closed. The loss of your accounts receivable records in a fire or from an act of vandalism would make it difficult for you to reconstruct your patient's financial records. Accounts receivable insurance to protect against losses from fire, theft, and vandalism may also be purchased (see Buying Insurance, p. 147).

Fire Safety

You should invest in a small fire extinguisher for your office. Fire extinguishers are classified on the basis of the types of fires that they can extinguish. There are three classifications of fires. *Class A* fires involve wood, plastic, paper, and cloth; *Class B* fires involve flammable liquids and grease; and *Class C* fires involve electrical equipment. Fire extinguishers may carry four classifications.

1. Class A contains water and is adequate for fighting class A fires.
2. Class AB contains a chemical foam for fighting classes A and B fires; it is not satisfactory for electrical fires.
3. Class BC contains a dry chemical for fighting classes B and C fires but is inadequate for fires involving wood, plastic, paper, and cloth.
4. Class ABC has a dry chemical mixture that is satisfactory for fighting all three classes of fires.

You should buy a class ABC fire extinguisher with at least five pounds of extinguishing material in it. The extinguisher should be manufactured with a pressure gauge on top so that you can periodically check the extinguisher to see if it is full and has not leaked its contents. The triggering mechanism should be secured with a removable pin and the extinguisher should come with a support to allow you to hang it in a convenient location. An adequate fire extinguisher may be purchased for less than fifty dollars.

When you purchase your waste receptacles you should also consider buying receptacles that are fire resistant. You should also consider installing a smoke and fire alarm system in your office. The installation of such a system may also reduce your fire insurance rate.

Informational Signs in Your Office

Attractive informational signs can be useful in your office. Examples of such signs include: "Be Considerate of Other Patients—No Smoking Please," "Please Register with the Receptionist Upon Entering," and "Fees Are Due and Payable Upon Completion of Your Visit—Any Other Arrangements Must be Made in Advance."

Many informational signs are mass produced and available from medical printing companies, such as Colwell, 201 Kenyon Road, Champaign, Illinois 61820 (800-637-1140), and Medical Arts Press, 3440 Winnetka Avenue, North, Minneapolis, Minnesota 55427 (612-545-3200) (see Appendix 24).

Your own custom designed informational signs may be manufactured by either the aforementioned companies or by your local office supply company.

Rubber Stamps and Labels

Your office aides will find it convenient to have custom made rubber stamps available for various purposes. These stamps are inexpensive and can be purchased from your local office supply company. Examples of some of the types of rubber stamps you should have available include

1. Rubber stamp with your name and office address
2. Rubber stamp for endorsing checks specifying "for deposit only," along with your bank account or savings account number
3. Rubber stamp for patient identification to be stamped on the endorsement side of the patient's check (see Receiving a Worthless Check, p. 144)
4. Rubber stamp specifying "benefits assigned" (see Insurance Claims, p. 109)
5. Rubber stamps for use on end-of-the-month statements for patient accounts that are delinquent (see Collecting Delinquent Accounts, p. 193)

As your practice grows and you develop your own business office routines, you will find other needs for rubber stamps.

Pressure sensitive, adhesive-backed labels are also a convenience to have and to place on various types of documents. These may include labels for overdue accounts; insurance billing, deduction, and rejection labels; and labels that relate to Medicare insurance. These may also be purchased from your local office supply company or from one of several firms that specialize in producing these types of labels.

Colwell Co.
201 Kenyon Rd.
Champaign, IL 61820
800-637-1140

United Ad Label
10035 S. Greenleaf Ave.
P. O. Box 2165
Whittier, CA 90610
213-944-7945

Medical Arts Press
3440 Winnetka Ave., North
Minneapolis, MN 55427
612-545-3200

Reference Books for Your Front Office

The following are a few suggested references to keep in your front office:

1. A standard English dictionary, such as *Webster's New Collegiate Dictionary,* G. & C. Merriam Company, Springfield, Massachusetts.
2. A standard medical dictionary, such as *Dorland's Illustrated Medical Dictionary,* W. B. Saunders Company, Philadelphia, Pennsylvania.
3. A medical secretarial handbook, such as *Webster's Medical Office Handbook,* G. & C. Merriam Company, Springfield, Massachusetts.
4. A book on disease classifications, such as *International Classification of Diseases* (ICDA). A copy of this reference may be obtained from the Superintendent of Documents, United States Government Printing Office, Washington, D.C. 20402.
5. The *Physicians' Desk Reference.* A free copy of the *Physicians' Desk Reference* may be obtained by writing to *Physicians' Desk Reference,* c/o Medical Economics, Oradell, New Jersey 07649.
6. *National Zip Code and Post Office Directory.* A copy of this reference may be obtained from the Superintendent of Documents, United States Gov-

ernment Printing Office, Washington, D.C. 20402, or in any of the 27 government printing office book stores in 20 major cities (see Appendix 34). The cost of this reference was two dollars per copy in 1982.

Pharmaceutical Company Representatives

Pharmaceutical company representatives will come to your office to acquaint you with their company's products. These pharmaceutical company representatives provide an important and valuable service. They will acquaint you with the newest drugs coming on the market and review with you the indications, side effects, and experimental data related to the new product.

Pharmaceutical company representatives should be seen in your office by appointment only. Your office aide should give a pharmaceutical company representative a ten- to fifteen-minute appointment. Some physicians have their office aides schedule appointments for pharmaceutical company representatives only on certain days of the week or during certain hours of the day. You should offer pharmaceutical company representatives the same courtesy that you would offer a patient and see them promptly so that they do not waste their day sitting in your reception room.

You should try to limit the number of pharmaceutical company representatives that you see in any one day. Emphasize that you are only interested in new products or in new uses for old products. A biweekly visit from a pharmaceutical company representative to tell you how wonderful his antibiotic may be is time consuming, and unless you just enjoy chatting about sports, hunting, the stock market, or current events with a particularly personable representative, you should try to limit these visits.

Pharmaceutical representatives will often leave samples of their company's products for you to give to your patients. These samples should be stored alphabetically in a locked storage closet. Periodically your office personnel should go through the medication and discard those that are outdated. Your practice habits will inevitably make you favor certain drugs in the treatment of diseases. It is obviously the role of the pharmaceutical representative to try to influence your practice habits in favor of one company's drugs.

If you have not used a drug that has been on your drug storage shelf for six months, you should consider discarding the drug to eliminate future storage problems. Pharmaceutical representatives should be asked not to leave excessive amounts of samples because of limitations of storage space.

Pharmaceutical companies also provide another excellent service by distributing free literature for patient education. Some of the best literature about common diseases can be obtained without cost from your pharmaceutical company representative. These include such things as diet manuals, booklets about control of hypertension, as well as other common disease entities like diverticulosis, peptic ulcer disease, heart disease, and reflux esophagitis (see also Patient Education, p. 117).

Within the last few years a number of pharmaceutical companies have developed slide presentations, movies, and programmed instruction for both patient and physician education.

Used properly, your pharmaceutical company representative can be a valuable source of free information making your practice easier, communications skills with your patients greater, and your own fund of knowledge about new drugs wider.

Handling the Mail

When your office aide receives the daily mail it may be separated into various categories.

1. *Advertising material and samples.* You should instruct your office aide regarding your policy for reviewing this type of mail. You may establish a schedule to review such mail once a week or twice a month or at some other convenient interval.
2. *General mail (sealed and sent first class).* Your office aide should open all of this mail. If the mail is from a patient, your aide should check the patient's address to verify that your records con-

tain the latest address information. The envelope should be attached to its contents to assure a proper return address when you dictate any return correspondence.

3. *First class (marked "personal")*. Unless you instruct your office aide differently, all mail marked "personal" should be put on your desk unopened.
4. *Invoices*. Your office aide may review the various items of indebtedness received from various firms and individuals for supplies, equipment, and services. You should spot-check bills of indebtedness at the time the bill is received in the mail or at the time your office aide presents a check to you for your signature when the office bills are routinely paid. By spot-checking you will remain aware of payments for various kinds of expenses.

3. Personnel Management

Hiring Help

To run a successful office you will need skilled personnel to help you. You may need a registered nurse, a licensed practical nurse, a laboratory x-ray technician, or skilled business office personnel.

1. *Where to find office personnel.* Here are a few suggestions how to find office aides.

   a. Advertise in the want ads of your local newspaper.
   b. Call the medical society of your community and inquire if a list of applicants for office jobs is available.
   c. Contact the larger, professional medical groups in your community and talk to each group's business manager, if it has one. Frequently, larger groups have a list of applicants on file to fill future job vacancies.
   d. Contact the personnel department of the local hospitals. These departments have applications on file for all types of personnel. It is not advisable, however, to "steal" the currently employed hospital personnel for your office.
   e. Contact an employment agency that may be willing to advertise or screen applicants for you.
   f. Check with technical schools, business schools, junior colleges, and nursing schools in the area, as well as laboratory and x-ray technician programs, and professional assistant programs.
   g. Contact the principal of the local high school or the teacher of the high school business course. Either of them may be able to identify a skilled student coming out of high school who is looking for a job in a professional office.

2. *How to screen for office aides.* If you are advertising in the newspaper, have the applicant answer by sending a resumé and a handwritten cover letter to a post office box. You can learn

a great deal about the applicant's training, formal education, and command of language from the way the resumé and cover letter are written. The applicant who has bad handwriting or a poor command of language should not be considered as a possible employee regardless of experience or training. It is courteous to call or send a rejection letter to all applicants who are not selected for the job. You should thank the applicant for taking the time and trouble to apply. You should state that another more qualified applicant has been selected.

3. *What kind of office aides?* There are many successful offices that have hired employees with no formal, specialized business office or nursing training. Your type of practice and the duties required by the personnel within the office will dictate the degree of specialty training that your personnel must have. When you start your practice, try to hire one assistant who can serve as a jack of all trades (your secretary, typist, receptionist, bookkeeper, and nursing assistant). As your practice grows you will add more help, allowing for a more specialized division of labor.
4. *The employment interview.* Contact by phone or mail those applicants who appear promising as potential employees for the job opening. Have these applicants complete a formal application and arrange an interview. You must be careful that your job application and interview do not violate the Federal Employment Practice Act. The basic law is contained in the 1964 Civil Rights Act (Public Law 88-352, Title VII) amended by the 1972 Equal Employment Opportunities Act. It outlaws job discrimination on the basis of race, color, sex, religion and national origin. This specific law is designed for employers with fifteen or more employees. The 1967 Age Discrimination Act, as amended in 1978, outlaws bias in the forty- to seventy-year age category. This act is designed for those employers with twenty-five or more employees. Even if you hire less than fifteen employees, the 1964 Civil Rights Act (Title VI, sec. 601) prohibits job discrimination in all programs or activities that re-

ceive federal aid. Since your office will be a recipient of Medicare and Medicaid funds, you must comply with this federal law. There are also state laws against job discrimination that are similar to the federal laws.

You should contact your state Department of Labor and familiarize yourself with these laws against discrimination. Usually state laws provide that employers cannot discriminate on the basis of physical or mental handicaps, weight, gender, or support of dependents unless such factors directly interfere with job performance. A number of job application forms have been prepared by business system companies that are acceptable and do not violate the federal laws. An example of such a job application appears in Figure 5.

At the time of the interview a great deal of knowledge can be obtained by judging the applicant's personal appearance, especially from aspects of personal hygiene such as hair grooming and care of fingernails. The applicant's voice, poise, and mannerisms are all important and may be readily assessed during the personal interview. Obviously most applicants are nervous and should not be judged solely on these factors. Key questions to ask during the personal interview include

a. Why does the applicant want to work in a professional office?
b. Why did the applicant leave his or her last job?
c. Why does the applicant feel particularly qualified to fill the position in your office?

You should allow the applicant time at the end of the interview to ask questions. If the applicant is joining your established staff of employees, give your current staff a chance to interview the applicant. Since your current staff will be working most closely with the applicant in the office, their impressions about a new applicant may be valuable in helping you select a new employee.

5. *Job description.* It is important to tell the applicant about the job during the job interview.

Classification ______________________
(Not to be Filled in by Applicant)

Date ______________________

APPLICATION FOR EMPLOYMENT

Name ______________________ Soc. Sec. No. ______________ Phone No. ______________
(Last) (First) (Middle)

Address ______________________ Birth Date ______________
(No.) (Street) (City) (State)

Spouse's name ______________ No. & ages of Children ______________ Other dependents ______________

List any friends or relatives in our employ ______________________

What transportation can you use to get to and from work? ______________________

Are you applying for: ______ full time ______ part time ______ temporary ______ summer

EDUCATION RECORD	Name and Place	From		To		Did you Graduate?	Course
Type of School		Mo.	Yr.	Mo.	Yr.		
Last Grammar or Jr. H.S.							
Last High or Prep. School							
College or University							
Other							

EXPERIENCE—PLEASE ACCOUNT FOR ALL TIME SINCE LEAVING SCHOOL—LIST LAST EMPLOYER FIRST

Firm Name	Place	Your Position	Dept. No.	Supervisor	From		To		Salary or Wages	Reason for Leaving
					Mo.	Yr.	Mo.	Yr.		

PLEASE COMPLETE REVERSE SIDE OF THIS SHEET

THIS COMPANY DOES NOT DISCRIMINATE ON THE BASIS OF AGE, SEX OR NATIONAL ORIGIN

Figure 5. Sample application for employment. (Courtesy of the Colwell Company, Champaign, Ill.)

(Ask for additional sheets if needed)

MILITARY RECORD

Service Army, Navy, etc.	Branch Infantry, etc.	Primary Duty	From		To		Special Service Training Mechanics, Military Police, etc.
			Mo.	Yr.	Mo.	Yr.	

What type of work do you prefer? ______

When could you start to work? ______ What monthly salary would you consider to start? ______

Give name, address, and business of each of two references:
(No relatives, but at least one former employer)

What special equipment have you used?

Describe previous experience you believe will help you in employment with us. ______

What are your hobbies? ______

Do you have any chronic ailments or other physical limitations which preclude you from performing certain kinds of work? ______

How many days have you been ill during the past two years? ______

Have you ever been hospital confined? ______ Where? ______ When? ______ Why? ______

Are you willing to submit to a medical examination? ______ Have you ever had any kind of industrial accident or occupational disease? ______

Have you ever been convicted of a felony? ______ Where? ______ When? ______

Would you agree to a personal investigation for security purposes? ______

______
(Signature of Applicant)

Interviewed by: ______ Date ______

This Application For Employment is prepared for use throughout the United States. The Colwell Company assumes no responsibility for the inclusion of any questions which, when asked by the employer of the job applicant, may violate state and/or federal law.

Figure 5. (Continued)

If you have already prepared an office manual outlining the job, you may ask the applicant to read it. Otherwise, you should present a brief sketch of the duties required, benefits paid, and general office policies.

When you hire a new office aide it is helpful to explain not only the primary responsibilities, but those duties he or she will be expected to perform when a co-worker is absent. You should also give the applicant a fair appraisal of the number of hours of work per week the job entails.

6. *Wages.* Find out from other physicians in the community and from your local hospitals what the going rate of payment is for office personnel and skilled nursing personnel. You do not have to pay the "top dollar" in town; on the other hand, you will not hire or keep good personnel by being the cheapest.

   The United States Department of Labor has statistics available that may assist you in establishing rates of pay. You may obtain from the Bureau of Labor Statistics the median weekly earnings of specific government job titles (see Appendix 21).

Title	*Corresponding Government Job Classification*
Office manager	Secretary, class A
Appointment secretary	Secretary, class B
Private secretary	Typist, class B
File clerk	File clerk, class C
Bookkeeper	Accounting clerk, class B

7. *Educational benefits.* Consider budgeting a specific amount of your employees' payroll for their continuing education. A figure commonly quoted is between 5 and 7 percent. The money may be used to reimburse your employees for convention expenses, teaching aids, filmstrips, books, and continuing education courses to improve their office skills.
8. *Working hours.* Full-time employees should be expected to work a forty-hour week. Part-time employees will work some percentage of a forty-hour week; for example, twenty hours per

week for a half-time employee, or ten hours per week for a quarter-time employee.

The Fair Labor Standards Act (United States Code Annotated, Title 29, sec. 201, et seq.) establishes the guidelines for paying minimum wages and overtime. Executive, administrative, and professional employees are exempt from minimum wage and overtime standards. The United States Department of Labor has specific regulations defining the meaning of executive, administrative, and professional employees. The regulations specify the level of administrative responsibility that must be given to an employee to qualify for wage and overtime exemption. Merely assigning a perfunctory title to an employee will not qualify the job for the exemption.

The Fair Labor Standards Act is explicit about paying non-exempt office workers 1½ times their salary for hours worked in excess of forty hours per week. The act does not allow averaging of hours over two or more weeks. For example, an employee who works thirty hours one week and fifty hours the next week must receive overtime pay for the hours worked beyond forty hours in the second week. You should be aware of those things that the Fair Labor Standards Act does *not* require.

a. Vacation pay
b. Severance pay
c. Discharge notices
d. Days off for holidays
e. Payment of overtime for working on Saturday, Sunday, or holidays

Two free booklets are available describing the requirements of the Fair Labor Standards Act: *Overtime Compensation Under the Fair Labor Standards Act (W. H. publication 1325)*, and *Records to be Kept by Employers Under the Fair Labor Standards Act of 1938, as amended.* These publications may be obtained from your local field office of the United States Department of Labor, or from the United States Department of Labor, Employee's Standards Administration, 200

Constitution Avenue, NW, Washington, D.C. 20210 (202-523-6191).

Although you, as the employer, may have a doctor's day off or afternoon off for yourself, this same practice need not be extended to your office aides. The physician's time out of the office should be used by office aides to catch up on insurance, billings, collection calls, restocking rooms with usable supplies, and other office tasks that are best done when patients are not being seen in the office.

9. *Probationary periods*. Make it clear to your new employees that the first 90 to 120 days (depending on your office policy) of employment constitute a probationary period. This period provides your new office aide time to evaluate the work and time to adjust to the work environment. It also provides you, the employer, the opportunity to see if the employee can perform the skills required. One advantage of formally defining a probationary period is that if you are dissatisfied with the employee's performance and you terminate your office aide's employment, your office will not have to pay unemployment compensation benefits that may be claimed by your unemployed aide and charged against your office's contribution to the unemployment compensation fund.

   Most states require that you contribute to an unemployment compensation fund based on your annual employee payroll and the claims made against your contributions by unemployed office workers. A formal declaration of a probationary period protects you against charges against your contributions to the unemployment compensation fund.

10. *Time off*

    a. *Holidays*. Most doctors' offices provide for six paid holidays. By custom these holidays are New Year's Day, Memorial Day, July 4th, Labor Day, Thanksgiving, and Christmas. If a holiday falls on a weekend, it is customary for you and your office staff to decide whether to take off the Friday before or the Monday after the holiday. Many doctors also close their offices early on Christmas Eve, New Year's Eve, and Thanksgiving Eve, since their practices tend to slow down on those days.

b. *Vacations.* It is common practice for a doctor to give full-time employees five paid days of vacation during the first year of employment. In the second, third, fourth, and fifth years of full-time employment, ten paid vacation days would be considered appropriate. Full-time employees who have worked six to nine years may be offered fifteen paid vacation days, and full-time employees with more than ten years' service might receive twenty paid vacation days.

c. *Sick leave and emergency leave.* Many physicians' offices provide for sick leave and emergency leave. The number of days may be set as a specific number of days per year or awarded as an accrued benefit based on the number of months of employment. For example, an employee may accrue one fully paid sick leave or emergency leave day for every three months of employment.

11. *Insurance benefits.* Insurance benefits have become routine for most offices. These include such benefits as

    a. *Health insurance.* A small office with a single practitioner and few employees may have difficulty establishing a group health insurance plan. An alternative is to provide a health insurance benefit by paying a cash reimbursement for medical and dental expenses. You may select a certain percent reimbursement for your employees based on their salary. For example, an employee earning $10,000 per year might receive 4 percent or $400 cash reimbursement for health related expenses. It would then be the employee's responsibility to fund insurance for hospitalization, a major medical policy, or other special medical coverage. The employee is usually required to provide some documentation that a medical, dental, or insurance expense has been paid in full to collect the allocated reimbursement.

b. *Life insurance and disability income insurance.* These insurance benefits are not mandatory benefits given to employees of unincorporated practices. However, these insurance benefits may be quite inexpensive if obtained through some of the group plans offered by medical associations, and they can be an extra benefit offered by your office. If you incorporate your practice, life and disability insurance may become significant fringe benefits for both you and the other corporate employees. Your corporation may pay for certain types of qualified life insurance plans and disability income insurance, however it is mandatory to provide a comparable benefit for all full-time employees.

c. *Workers' Compensation insurance.* As an employer you may be required to pay Workers' Compensation insurance. The laws regulating Workers' Compensation insurance vary from state to state. You should write to your state's regulatory agency to receive information regarding your state's requirements for Workers' Compensation insurance (see Appendix 22).

12. *Pay schedule.* At the time that you hire an office aide you should describe your office pay schedule. Some offices pay on a weekly basis, but most pay either on the fifteenth and thirtieth of the month or on a biweekly basis. Most office workers find it more convenient for their personal financial budgeting to be paid weekly or biweekly rather than monthly. You should consider paying your office personnel on an hourly basis rather than offering monthly salary. There are some recognized disadvantages to paying your office personnel a monthly salary rather than on an hourly basis. Personnel working on a monthly salary basis have a tendency to come in later, leave earlier, take longer lunch hours, and take more time off from their daily

schedule for personal reasons than individuals paid on an hourly basis. Regardless of how you pay your personnel, the United States Department of Labor requires that accurate time records be kept for all office employees. If your employees work on an hourly basis, an inexpensive time clock can be installed in your office. Most business supply companies sell time clocks and the necessary time cards.

13. *Grounds for dismissal.* The major grounds for dismissal should be discussed with your employees at the time they are hired. These reasons might include the following:

    a. Incompetence
    b. Conviction of a major crime (felony)
    c. Repeated or gross negligence in the performance of duty
    d. Insubordination
    e. Unjustified absenteeism
    f. Embezzlement of office money
    g. Disorderly or unprofessional conduct
    h. Working under the influence of alcohol
    i. Falsification of information on an employment application
    j. Destruction of office equipment
    k. Falsification of time records
    l. Misuse of controlled substances
    m. Violation of confidential information

    There are state and federal laws dealing with discrimination in dismissal of employees. For example, federal laws prohibit the dismissal of an employee solely on the basis of race, sex, religion, national origin, or age if the employee is over forty. If you have a question regarding possible discrimination and dismissal of an employee you should contact the Equal Employment Opportunity Commission of the federal government or of the state in which you practice.

14. *Reference Checks.* Your employment application form will require the prospective employee to list personal references as well as to give a previous job history. Make a practice to check all references given by the prospective em-

ployee. Bear in mind that personal references listed by the employee will tend to include individuals favorably disposed to the applicant. Contact all of your prospective employee's previous employers. Talk to the prospective employee's previous supervisor and discuss the following information, if possible:

a. Dates of employment
b. Description of the position held including duties, skills, and contact with the general public
c. Starting and ending salaries
d. The applicant's ability to cooperate with co-workers
e. The applicant's attendance and health record
f. The applicant's major strengths and weaknesses
g. The reason the applicant left the previous place of employment
h. Whether the supervisor would rehire the applicant

15. *Miscellaneous office policies and procedures.* Other items that you might consider discussing at the time of your initial hiring include uniform allowances, time off for lunch, office policies regarding wearing perfume, jewelry, and make-up, and confidentiality of office matters.
16. *Office policy manuals.* An office policy manual will help you outline for new employees all of your basic office guidelines. It also provides a set of rules to which both new and old employees can refer for answers to questions related to most office policy matters. It is best to outline your office policies in advance rather than make policy as you go (see Appendix 38).

Advertising for Employee Help

When you advertise to fill a vacancy in your office personnel, you may wish to place a want ad in your local newspaper. The want ad should contain the following information:

1. The title of the vacant position; for example, medical assistant, secretary–receptionist, licensed

practical nurse, registered nurse, or bookkeeper

2. The amount of experience required; for example, no experience required or some experience required
3. The duties of the job; for example, for reception, for answering the telephone, for medical transcription, or for bookkeeping
4. The hours required; for example, part-time, full-time, evenings, Saturdays, or overtime
5. Request for a resumé with references
6. Request for a handwritten cover letter

The want ad should conclude by listing a box number at the newspaper office. For a small additional fee, most newspaper advertising departments provide a service allowing readers to respond to a box number. A sample of a want ad for a medical assistant might read:

> Medical assistant: Previous doctor's office or hospital experience desired. Duties include reception, answering the telephone, and medical transcription. Will offer training. Forty-hour week with no evenings, Saturdays, or overtime required. Send a typewritten resumé with references and handwritten cover letter to *The Daily Herald,* P. O. Box 123.

Hiring Relatives

Generally speaking, it is not recommended that you use relatives in your office as part of your office staff. Do not hire someone you may be unable to fire. There are, of course, exceptions. If you do hire relatives, you must take into account the following economic considerations:

1. Be able to justify that the family member employed has the training and can do the work the job requires. For example, you cannot have your spouse come into your office two hours each month to help you get out the end-of-the-month bills and pay your spouse a $10,000 a year salary.
2. Be able to justify your family member's salary deduction as a business expense. Be able to prove that the services described have actually been performed. The Internal Revenue Service (IRS) may deny you a business expense deduction for a family member if it concludes that the deduc-

tion is an effort to siphon off practice profits for your family member's support.

3. Keep a detailed record or a time card for hours worked by any family member employee to show the IRS if you are audited.
4. Treat family member employees like all other employees. You must take out withholding tax from a family member employee's paycheck. A deduction for Social Security must be made, and as the employer, you must make an equal contribution to the Social Security system.
5. If you are married and if you hire your spouse to work in your office, The Economic Recovery Tax Act of 1981 provides for certain tax benefits.

   a. You and your spouse may receive a tax credit on your joint income tax return in an amount up to $4,800 for the costs involved in the care of two or more dependents.
   b. You and your spouse may receive a tax credit on your joint income tax return for 1982 amounting to 5 percent, or a maximum of $1,500, of your spouse's income. In 1983 and thereafter, these figures will increase to 10 percent, or a maximum of $3,000.
   c. As a wage earner your spouse may contribute to an Individual Retirement Account (IRA) in an amount equal to 15 percent of yearly earned income, up to a maximum of $2,000. The amount invested in an IRA is sheltered from current taxes. If you are married and your spouse is not an employee of your office or otherwise employed, the Economic Recovery Tax Act still allows you to contribute to an IRA for both you and your spouse up to a maximum of $2,250 per year. Unmarried persons may contribute up to $2,000 per year to an IRA. The contribution may be made to an IRA even if you contribute to a corporate retirement plan (see Retirement Plans, p. 158).

Social Security Earnings Record

It is advisable for you and your employees to request a statement of your Social Security credits once a year. You can check your record to make sure your account has been properly credited. Government computers have been known to make mistakes and it is preferable to catch an error in the year that it occurs than to try to unscramble errors when you retire and file for your Social Security benefits.

You can receive a free statement of your Social Security credits by sending form 7004-P. C. to the Social Security Administration, Post Office Box 57, Baltimore, Maryland 21203 (301-792-7100). The Social Security administration form 7004-P. C. may be obtained from your local Social Security administration office.

End-of-the-Year Job Summary

You should consider providing your employees with an annual summary of their employment benefits. You are required to provide your employees with an annual accounting of retirement plan benefits if you are incorporated. You are also required to give them a W–2 form to file with their income tax in January of each year, showing their gross salaries and the Federal Withholding and Social Security taxes deducted from their salaries. A complete summary of benefits, however, might include both the information contained on the W–2 form and other information, including

1. Salary
2. Retirement plan contributions made by you or your corporation
3. Bonuses (if not already included in the salary computation)
4. Medical expense reimbursements or premiums paid for medical insurance
5. Disability insurance premiums
6. Life insurance premiums
7. Workers' compensation insurance premiums
8. Your contribution to the employee's Social Security account (equivalent to the Social Security deduction the employee pays)
9. Estimated cost of refreshments (e.g., colas, coffee)

10. Payments for continuing education, conventions, and seminars
11. Uniform allowances
12. Unemployment taxes
13. Other

The benefit summary gives your employees a better idea of the monetary value of their jobs. It also serves as a point of reference for your employees should they compare their present jobs with other job opportunities that they might consider.

Caring for Your Office Aides

You should encourage your staff to have their own family physicians. You may be willing to attend to your office staff's minor ailments and give temporary health advice, and perhaps even prescribe mild analgesics, antiemetics, antacids, or antidiarrheal agents. Your office aides should seek other professional advice for major or recurrent illnesses and long-term health care.

Emergency Equipment and Emergency Training

Every medical office should have some basic cardiopulmonary resuscitation equipment. An oropharyngeal airway and a few cardiac drugs may be all that your office requires. If you are seeing large numbers of cardiology patients or doing stress electrocardiograms, you should consider purchasing a more sophisticated cardiopulmonary resuscitation system, including defibrillation equipment.

Banyan International, 2118 East Interstate 20, Post Office Box 1779, Abilene, Texas 79604 (915-677-1874), is one company that makes a variety of resuscitation kits for office use. Their kits come with varying amounts of equipment. Most of the basic cardiopulmonary resuscitation drugs are included in the kits, such as sodium bicarbonate, epinephrine, calcium chloride, methoxamine hydrochloride, lidocaine, and calcium carbonate. These drugs, as well as disposable syringes, needles, and individual glass drug ampules are all supplied. An intravenous administration set is included along with intravenous solutions. The basic kits all contain Welch Allyn laryngoscopes with a light source plus endotracheal tubes and oropharyngeal airways. The most complete units contain portable oxygen delivery systems, resuscitators, and surgical equipment such as scalpels, sutures, and hemostats.

Banyan International emergency office equipment is conveniently packaged in a durable aluminum case. The approximate cost for these kits through local surgical supply companies in 1982 ranged from $230 for the simplest kit to $630 for the most complete kit with oxygen delivery systems and surgical instruments.

All office personnel should be encouraged and given the opportunity to attend training courses in cardiopulmonary resuscitation. This training should be offered to your front office aides as well as to your skilled nursing personnel. Cardiopulmonary resuscitation refresher courses are frequently sponsored by local hospitals, the American Heart Association, medical schools, or the local Red Cross agency. If there is no course available in your community, you should encourage one of the local cardiologists to sponsor such a course. The Joint Commission on Accreditation of Hospitals also encourages every physician, regardless of specialty, to receive instruction on cardiopulmonary resuscitation followed by yearly refresher courses.

It Pays to Be a Good Boss

Man does not live by bread alone, nor by paychecks alone. Your aides need encouragement and praise from you when it is warranted. They need to be told they are doing a good job and rewarded, not just with their paychecks but with other niceties. Most offices offer standard fringe benefits as previously discussed (see Hiring Help, p. 65). You should consider offering little extras that will make your office special. These extras do not have to be costly, yet they can give your office staff an esprit de corps that will make your life more pleasant and your office a happier environment in which to work. Most of the little extras are deductible expenses for your practice and are worth more than their cost in keeping your employees happy. Consider the following:

1. Give your worthy office aides a bonus periodically.
2. Give your office aides a Christmas gift. Most employees prefer a little extra in their paycheck rather than a gift that may not be needed.
3. Buy soft drinks and snacks for your employees. If you provide this extra, you should periodically monitor your expenses to make sure this benefit is not abused.
4. Celebrate employee birthdays in your office. You should buy the refreshments.
5. If employees drive their own cars to run personal errands for you, reimburse them with a tank of gasoline occasionally.
6. Provide simple food preparation utensils in the office like a hot plate and a coffee maker. A more substantial extra would be a microwave oven.

4. Office Practice Management

Scheduling Your Office Appointments

When you begin your practice you will probably have only a few appointments scheduled each day. However, these appointments should be scheduled close together. As one person is entering your office another should be leaving so that you will get into the habit of planning your day efficiently and contending with a full schedule. The busy day and full schedule will soon become a reality.

The time it takes for a doctor to see scheduled patients may vary from doctor to doctor and from specialty to specialty. Some physicians will schedule six to eight patients per hour to be seen throughout the day while others will schedule only one or two new patients and a few followup appointments.

There are basically three types of scheduling methods that can be used in your office. The first method is called the *wave* system. In essence, the wave system is no system at all. No appointment scheduling is used and all patients are processed on a first come, first served basis. This system has the greatest potential for delaying patients the longest periods of time in your reception room. It also creates the most erratic patterns of patient flow for the doctor, with episodic peaks and lulls in workload.

The second method for scheduling patients is called the *stream* approach. Patients are scheduled at regular intervals according to an appointment log. Most appointment logs are divided into fifteen-minute time segments throughout the day. Patients are given appointments and are instructed to come into the office every fifteen minutes or in multiples of fifteen minutes. Patient appointments, however, rarely last exactly the time interval allocated on the appointment log (whether the time interval is ten, fifteen, or twenty minutes, or longer). Some patients require less time and others require more. In those instances when a patient is seen quickly, in less than the time period allocated on the appointment log, the physician's work pattern is interrupted during the interval before the next patient comes in. In those instances when the patient's care requires a longer period than the time allocated on the appointment log, the physician falls behind schedule. The stream approach, using fixed-interval appointment scheduling, rarely provides for optimal patient flow and utilization of physician time.

The most efficient method for scheduling patients is known as the *modified wave system*. The physician determines an hourly rate for seeing various types of patients. The appointment schedule is divided into hourly segments. The total number of patients who are to be seen in each hour's time is scheduled in clustered groups. One-half of the patients who the physician might see in an hour's time are scheduled on the hour. The remainder of the patients are scheduled at intervals throughout the hour with all of the patients scheduled within the first forty-five minutes of the hour.

For example, if four patients would ordinarily be seen by a physician from 9:00 to 10:00 A.M., these four patients would be scheduled so that two would be given a 9:00 appointment, the next a 9:15 appointment, and the last a 9:30 appointment. If the physician finishes seeing patients before the end of the hour, the remaining time may be used to dictate records, return telephone calls, take a coffee break, or catch up on reading. The modified wave approach reduces patient waiting time as well as lag time for a physician between patients.

Each doctor must set his or her own pace and style of practice. The following guidelines, however, will offer additional help in making your patient-flow smoother and your appointment schedule run on time.

1. Try to be on time. No appointment scheduling system can accommodate the physician who is habitually late.
2. Allow additional time in your schedule for predictably longer visits. Talkative patients should be given appointments at the end of the day.
3. Have patients who are being seen in your office for the first time arrive early to register.
4. Allow extra time in your schedule for doctors' calls and unavoidable interruptions as well as

emergency work-ins. Allowing time for emergency work-ins will keep you on time and will avoid the closed appointment book, a situation whereby critically ill patients are virtually screened out of your practice because your appointment book is filled by patients who have scheduled well in advance.

5. Consider scheduling all of the patients to be seen during the last hour of the day at the beginning of the last hour. In this way you can avoid delays caused by a late patient who may prevent you and your office staff from closing the office on time. If you finish seeing the last hour of patients ahead of schedule, you have an opportunity to leave the office early.
6. Give salespeople and pharmaceutical company representatives an appointment to be seen in your office. Schedule such appointments on your appointment log the same as you would for a patient (see Pharmaceutical Company Representatives, p. 62).
7. Do not undermine your appointment schedule. The physician should direct all appointments through the scheduling secretary. Physicians should not tell a patient to come into the office without checking the appointment log to make sure that work-in time is available.
8. Call or send reminder notices to new patients to minimize the number of no shows.
9. See walk-in patients only after patients with appointments have been seen. Have such patients return at a specific scheduled appointment time, if possible.
10. Indicate in your office policy manual that you reserve the right to bill a patient for a cancelled appointment if your office is not notified at least twenty-four hours in advance.

Patient Reminders

You should develop a method to remind patients of their office appointments. There are several methods that can be used.

1. *Telephone reminders.* One of your office aides can call patients twenty-four to forty-eight hours

in advance of the patient's appointment and remind the patient about the appointment. This system is effective but time consuming if you have a large number of patients to contact. In addition, your aides may not be able to reach your patient by telephone during your normal office hours.

2. *Appointment cards*. When patients leave your office, your aide may give them a printed appointment reminder. The reminder may be printed on the charge slip that the patient receives after an office visit or it may be printed on the reverse side of a business card (see Pegboard Accounting, p. 133). Eyecatching reminder notices can be made with adhesive for patients to attach to a mirror or bulletin board.
3. *Mailed reminder notices*. A mailed reminder notice is recommended for the doctor who schedules patient appointments far in advance. However, it is considered a violation of medical ethics to solicit a patient's return to your office. If you wish to use a mailed reminder notice ask patients when they leave your office if they wish to receive reminder notices. Print your reminders with a message stating "At your request, we are reminding you of your appointment scheduled for ____________________ at ________ A.M. / P.M. If you are unable to keep this appointment, please call the office at least 24 hours in advance." Some doctor's offices have the patient fill out his name and address on the front of a postcard with the aforementioned message. The patient's own writing quickly catches his eye, and the card makes an effective reminder that falls well within the bounds of medical ethics.

Telephone Reception by Your Office Aide

Your telephone receptionist should be friendly, sympathetic, relaxed, and unhurried when conversing with patients. When talking to a new patient making an appointment, the aide should obtain the patient's name, address, telephone number, age, and the type of problem that concerns the patient. A printed form for this type of information can be designed and kept next to your telephones. Most business office supply companies have standard telephone message forms that may be used.

1. *Explanation of office policies.* Some doctors have their receptionists explain their office polices to the patient at the time that the patient makes an initial appointment. The receptionist may discuss such things as initial office fees, records and drugs that the patient should bring along, and the doctor's office hours. After a patient has made an initial office appointment you should consider having your office aide send the patient a written booklet outlining your office policies. The booklet might include such things as

    a. Office hours
    b. Procedure for scheduling and breaking appointments
    c. Handling emergencies
    d. Daytime and after-hour telephone numbers
    e. Telephone consultation fees, if any
    f. Filling prescriptions and refills
    g. Policy regarding filing of insurance
    h. Policy for handling bills for laboratory testing
    i. Calling for test results
    j. Policy regarding hospitalization
    k. Professional fees
    l. Monthly billing procedure
    m. Methods of payment
    n. Housecalls
    o. Evening, weekend, and holiday coverage
    p. Other

    The American Medical Association has an inexpensive pamphlet entitled *Preparing a Patient Information Booklet* that is an excellent guide. Copies may be obtained from the American Medical Association, Order Department, OP-441, Post Office Box 821, Monroe, Wisconsin 53566.

    You might also consider sending the patient your initial history questionaire or registration form along with a map to your office before the first office visit (see Preparing a Medical History Form, p. 89).

2. *Screening telephone calls.* Your telephone recep-

tionist should learn to screen your office telephone calls. Make it clear to your office aide which telephone calls you will accept at the time the call is placed and which calls you will return at the end of your office hours.

a. *Emergency calls.* Educate your office aides about symptoms that usually constitute an emergency, such as high fever, severe abdominal pain, chest pain, shortness of breath, and excess bleeding. You should be interrupted immediately to take these calls.
b. *Physician calls.* It is accepted medical etiquette to accept all physician calls at the time that the call is received, if possible. Have your office aides routinely inquire whether the call is in reference to an established patient so that the patient's file can be pulled and be in front of you when the case is discussed. Instruct your office aides to wait for the calling physician to come to the telephone before paging you for the call. You should also be prepared to wait a few minutes for another physician to come to the telephone when you are placing the call.
c. *Family calls.* You should leave instructions with your office aides regarding your policy for accepting personal family calls. Most physicians will accept telephone calls immediately from their families. Family members should also be asked not to call you during office hours unless it is absolutely necessary.
d. *Business calls.* You should leave instructions for your office aides to interrupt you for calls from only certain specified business associates. For example, you might accept calls from your broker, accountant, or attorney, but instruct your office aides to take messages from all other business callers and you will return their calls at the end of your office hours.
e. *Hospital calls.* Many hospital calls from the nursing staff can be screened by your office aides. Make sure that your office aides impress on the nurse placing the call that if the matter is important and cannot be relayed as a message to you that you can be interrupted. Otherwise the nurse should be told that you

will return the call at the next convenient break in your office hours.

Preparing a Medical History Form

The preparation of a medical history form will save you and your office aides a great deal of time during the process of registering new patients and taking their initial histories. Your history form may range from a few questions to several hundred questions, depending on your type of practice and the amount of information you wish to obtain. Some general guidelines will help you develop your history form (Fig. 6).

1. Have your form printed in large, easy-to-read type.
2. Design your medical history form so that the average patient can complete it in less than fifteen minutes. If patients are expected to complete the form in your office as part of the registration process, a complicated form requiring more than fifteen minutes to complete will frequently delay processing the patient's records, thereby putting you behind in your office schedule.
3. Try to send the medical history form to your patients in advance of the initial office visit. This will allow the patient time to fill out the form in detail at home, thereby avoiding possible delays in registration when the patient comes to the office.
4. Leave a supply of your medical history forms at the hospitals where you practice. Have new patients who you have not seen in the office and patients who you are seeing in consultation complete your medical history form. This procedure will expedite evaluation of the patient's case history and allow you to concentrate on the patient's major presenting medical problem.
5. Design your medical history form so that the questions are simple and not ambiguous. Avoid compound questions such as: Do you frequently suffer from nausea, vomiting, and abdominal pain? It is preferable to ask: Do you suffer from nausea? Yes ___ No___ If yes, specify how often ______. Do you have abdominal pain? Yes ___ No ___ If yes, specify how often __________.

DEAN C. KRAMER, M.D., P.A.
6628 N.W. 9TH BOULEVARD
GAINESVILLE, FLORIDA 32605
TELEPHONE (904) 373-6736

Dear Patient:

The following questions are designed to obtain some general information about your medical problems. As a result of answering these questions it is intended that more time will be available for detailed discussion of your major medical problems.

Please complete the front and back of each side of all pages.

OFFICE PATIENTS

Your appointment is scheduled for ______________________ at ______ a.m. Please complete this form and bring it with you at the time of your appointment. We ask that you kindly arrive thirty (30) minutes before the above scheduled time so that you may register with the receptionist and have your records prepared.

Please do **not** eat or drink anything after midnight on the night before your office appointment. Please bring all of your prescription medications with you.

HOSPITAL PATIENTS

If this history form was given to you in the hospital, please complete all sections **except** "Insurance Information" and return it immediately to the nurse.

PATIENT INFORMATION *(Please print or type)*

Name: ______________________ Sex: Male [ ] Female [ ]

Address: ______________________ Age: __________

______________________ Date of Birth: __________
(City) (State) (Zip)

Social Security Number: ______________ Home Phone: __________

Drivers License Number: ______________ Office Phone: __________

Present Employer: ______________________

Employer's Address: ______________________

Years employed by present employer: ________ Position or Title: __________

Spouse's Name: ______________________ Spouse's Age: __________

Spouse's Employer: ______________________

Spouse's Employer's Address: ______________________

Spouse's Employer's Phone: ______________ Spouse's Title: __________

Nearest Friend or Relative Not Living With You: ______________________

Address: ______________________ Telephone: __________

Relationship: ______________________

Figure 6. Medical history form.

Marital Status: [ ]single, [ ]married, [ ]widowed, [ ]separated, [ ]divorced

Person responsible for payment of your professional fees: [ ]myself, [ ]other:

(indicate name, address, and telephone number): ____________________

____

Referred By: ____________________

List the names of all the doctors you have seen in the last two years and the reason why you have seen the doctor(s): ____________________

____

INSURANCE INFORMATION

(If this history form was given to you in the hospital, you may skip this section and proceed to the next section.)

Do you have hospitalization insurance? (check one) [ ] Yes [ ] No

Is your illness covered by Workers' Compensation Insurance? [ ] Yes [ ] No

If you have insurance coverage, please indicate the type(s):

[ ] Medicare........................Medicare Number: ____________________

[ ] Medicaid........................Medicaid Number: ____________________

[ ] Blue Cross-Blue Shield ....Contract Number: ____________________

[ ] Federal Blue Cross-Blue Shield ..Contract Number: ____________________

[ ] CHAMPUS

[ ] Other Insurance Coverage: (List below)

Name of company or companies and contract numbers: ____________________

____

____

MAJOR MEDICAL PROBLEM

Describe briefly the major medical problem that bothers you the most. ____________________

____

____

____

PAST MEDICAL HISTORY

Serious past injuries: (describe the type of injury and approximate dates of occurrence)

____

Previous surgery: (place a check-mark (✓) in the box next to the type of surgery you have had and indicate the approximate date of the surgery)

[ ] Appendix ____________________ [ ] Hernia ____________________

[ ] Cataracts ____________________ [ ] Hysterectomy ____________________

[ ] Gallbladder ____________________ [ ] Stomach ulcer surgery ____________________

[ ] Hemorrhoids removed ____________________ [ ] Tonsils ____________________

[ ] Other surgery: ____________________

____

Figure 6. (Continued)

Place a check-mark (✓) in the box next to the illness or illnesses that you currently have or have had in the past:

[ ] Anemia	[ ] Gout	[ ] Mental illness
[ ] Arthritis	[ ] Heart attack	[ ] Nervous stomach
[ ] Asthma	[ ] Heart trouble	[ ] Rheumatic fever
[ ] Cancer	[ ] Hepatitis	[ ] Spastic colon
[ ] Cirrhosis	[ ] High blood pressure	[ ] Stomach ulcers
[ ] Emphysema	[ ] Kidney infections	[ ] Sugar diabetes
[ ] Gallstones	[ ] Kidney stones	[ ] Thyroid trouble
[ ] Glaucoma	[ ] Liver disease	[ ] Yellow jaundice

FAMILY HISTORY

Is your mother living? [ ] Yes [ ] No (cause of death ____________)

Is your father living? [ ] Yes [ ] No (cause of death ____________)

Have any family members either living or dead ever had any of the following diseases? If **yes,** place a check-mark (✓) in the box next to the illness. In the space next to the illness put the name of the family member or the initial code letter of the family member that had the illness. The following code initials may be used:

Mother [M]	Brother [B]	Aunt [A]
Father [F]	Child [C]	Uncle [U]
Sister [S]	Grandparent [GP]	Cousin [CS]

For example: If one of your grandparents and a cousin had tuberculosis:
[✓] tuberculosis GP, CS

	Family Member		Family Member
[ ] Cancer	____________	[ ] High blood pressure	____________
[ ] Colitis	____________	[ ] Kidney disease	____________
[ ] Diabetes	____________	[ ] Tuberculosis	____________
[ ] Epilepsy	____________	[ ] Ulcers	____________
[ ] Heart attack	____________	[ ]	____________

SOCIAL HISTORY AND HABITS

Place a check-mark (✓) in the box that most closely approximates how much of the following alcoholic beverages you average drinking **per week:**

Beer:	[ ] none [ ] 7 to 18 cans	[ ] one to six cans [ ] more than 18 cans
Wine:	[ ] none [ ] between 16 and 32 ounces	[ ] less than 16 ounces [ ] more than 32 ounces
Liquor (Scotch, Gin, etc.):	[ ] none [ ] between 16 and 32 ounces	[ ] less than 16 ounces [ ] more than 32 ounces

Figure 6. (Continued)

Place a check-mark (✓) in the box that most closely approximates how much cigarette smoking you average **each day:**

[ ] none [ ] less than a half pack [ ] more than a half pack but less than one pack

[ ] one to two packs [ ] more than two packs

Place a check-mark (✓) in the box that most closely approximates how many **years** you have been a cigarette smoker:

[ ] 1-5 years [ ] 6-10 years [ ] 11-15 years [ ] 16-25 years

[ ] more than 25 years

Place a check-mark (✓) in the box that most closely approximates how much of the following beverages you drink **each day:**

Coffee:	[ ] none	[ ] 1-3 cups or glasses	[ ] 4-10	[ ] more than 10
Tea:	[ ] none	[ ] 1-3 cups or glasses	[ ] 4-10	[ ] more than 10
Colas:	[ ] none	[ ] 1-3 bottles	[ ] 4-10	[ ] more than 10

Place a circle around the highest level you obtained in school:

none	1 2 3 4 5 6 7 8	9 10 11 12	1 2 3 4
	elementary	high school	college

Masters PhD. Other: ______________________

List below all the medications that you take regularly or have taken regularly in the last month (including aspirin products, vitamins, birth control pills, etc.):

PLEASE BRING YOUR PRESCRIPTION MEDICATIONS WITH YOU.

Drug	Drug Strength	How often you take the drug each day.	Length of time you have taken the drug.
Example: *Valium*	*5 mg*	*three times a day*	*six months*

Figure 6. (Continued)

REVIEW OF SYMPTOMS

List any drug allergies: ______________________________

Are you allergic to Penicillin? (check one) [ ] Yes [ ] No

What is your usual weight? ________ What was your approximate weight one year ago?____________ What is your present weight? ______________

	YES	NO
1. Have you gained five pounds or more in the last two months?	[ ]	[ ]
2. Have you lost five pounds or more in the last two months?	[ ]	[ ]
3. Are you frequently troubled with coughing?	[ ]	[ ]
4. Have you ever coughed up blood or blood streaked sputum?	[ ]	[ ]
5. Do you frequently get short of breath?	[ ]	[ ]
6. Have you recently had repeated episodes of chest pain?	[ ]	[ ]
7. Are you frequently bothered by stomach pains?	[ ]	[ ]
8. Do you frequently have "heartburn" or "indigestion"?	[ ]	[ ]
9. Have you recently been bothered by abdominal bloating, belching, distention, or gaseousness?	[ ]	[ ]
10. Are you frequently bothered by vomiting?	[ ]	[ ]
11. Have you ever vomited blood?	[ ]	[ ]
12. Have you ever passed blood in or on your stools?	[ ]	[ ]
13. Are you frequently bothered by diarrhea?	[ ]	[ ]
14. Are you frequently bothered by constipation?	[ ]	[ ]
15. Do you experience pain or burning when you urinate?	[ ]	[ ]
16. Do you have difficulty getting your urinary stream started?	[ ]	[ ]
17. Do you awaken frequently during the night to urinate?	[ ]	[ ]
18. Do your joints frequently bother you?	[ ]	[ ]
19. Do you have frequent headaches?	[ ]	[ ]
20. Have you ever had a stroke, convulsion, fit, or paralysis?	[ ]	[ ]
21. Do you often feel scared or anxious?	[ ]	[ ]
22. Have you recently felt sad, depressed, or "down in the dumps"? ..	[ ]	[ ]
23. Have you recently had crying spells or felt like crying for no particular reason?	[ ]	[ ]
24. Do you feel tired and "worn out" most of the time?	[ ]	[ ]
25. WOMEN: Have you had a cervical "Paps" smear in the last two years?	[ ]	[ ]
26. WOMEN: Have you noticed any lumps in your breasts?	[ ]	[ ]

Figure 6. (Continued)

Constructing the Office Chart

1. *Preparing chart files.* The most commonly used chart container is a manila folder. These folders come in various sizes. The size generally selected for a doctor's office is a letter-sized manila folder for $8^1/_2$- by 11-inch stationery. You should select a heavy, durable folder for your office chart. Usually a file folder ranging from eleven- to fifteen-point thickness is adequate for most office charts. Manila folders can be purchased with

clasps, in various colors, and with a variety of material printed on the front of the folder, such as calendar years or sequential numbers. The file folders also come with a tab that extends beyond the margin of the folder for patient identification. The following is an inexpensive, successful filing system recommended for physicians using open shelf or lateral shelf filing:

a. Order manila, letter-sized, shelf filing folders, with full side cut and reinforced right edge in eleven- to fifteen-point thickness. It is unnecessary and expensive to obtain file folders in various colors.
b. Type the patient's name on a small gummed label with the last name first in capital letters. The patient's name identification label is attached to the side tab (see Fig. 7). All identification labels that are placed on the side tab of the chart should wrap around the edge so that they are visible from both sides of the file.
c. Color code the first two letters of the patient's last name (surname) and attach the letters to the side tab of the file folder beneath the patient's typed name. In practices with large numbers of files, the first three letters of the surname are color coded and attached to the side tab beneath the patient's name.
d. For patients with common surnames (e.g., Smith, Jones, or Brown), attach an additional color coded initial indicating the first letter of the patient's first name to the side tab of the file above the name identification label.
e. Attach a color coded tab above the patient's name bearing the last two digits of the year in which the patient last contacted your office.

2. *Chart materials.* The material within a patient's file should be assembled in chronological order. If the chart becomes bulky, it may be necessary to divide the chart into sections such as insurance, x-ray reports, office notes, correspondence, laboratory data, and electrocardiograms. Reports may vary in size and shape. To avoid losing odd-sized reports and to insure a neat and organized file, attach all odd-sized reports to an 8½- by

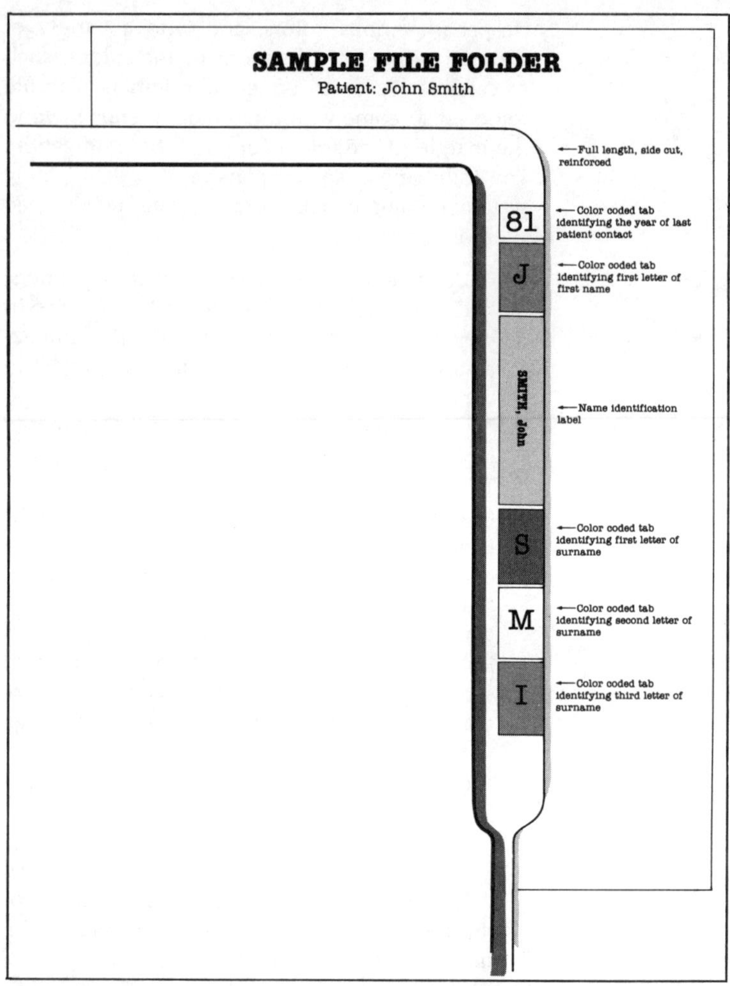

Figure 7. Sample file folder for patient John Smith.

11-inch sheet of paper. All papers in the patient's file should be identified with the patient's name and a date of entry. The patient's chart should contain all matters of medical relevance including

a. Ingoing and outgoing correspondence
b. Laboratory data
c. X-ray reports
d. Surgical reports

e. Consultant letters
f. Electrocardiograms
g. Insurance information
h. Hospital records
i. Records of every office contact

Dividing Files for Growth and Storage

As your practice grows, the number of patient files will grow. You must decide how to organize your files for growth and storage. There are several possible systems that can be used.

1. *The unit system.* In this system the new and old charts are all housed together in one large filing area. In a fast growing practice with a finite amount of filing space, the number of charts may rapidly outgrow the space for filing.
2. *The classified system.* In the classified system, patients' charts are filed according to their classification: active, inactive, and closed. With this system, some method must be used to establish criteria for the activity of the file in your office. Your office aides must review the files periodically to keep the classification up-to-date.
3. *The chronological–classified system.* In the chronological–classified system, a color coded label bearing the last two digits of the year is placed on the edge of the file each time a new patient file is made (see Constructing the office chart, p. 94). The same procedure is followed for established patients. Each time the patient returns to the practice (for an office visit, hospital admission, or consultation), the current color coded label is placed over the old label on the edge of the chart. Using this method your office aide can quickly scan your files and identify the year in which every patient was last seen.

   Files are purged according to your office policy by removing those charts for storage that do not have a color coded label within a specific time period. The purged charts are stored by the year in which the patient made his last office contact.

   This system requires the maintenance of a permanent identification file for all patients who have been seen since the beginning of your practice.

When a patient's file folder is returned to inactive status and placed in storage, an entry is made on the permanent identification card identifying the year in which the patient made his last contact with your office. If the patient returns several years later, the patient's permanent identification card can be reviewed to ascertain the year in which the old file was stored. When the file is retrieved from storage, a color coded label for the current year is placed on the file folder and the file is returned to the active files. This system works equally well for a numerical as well as an alphabetical file system. Before files are placed in storage, your office aide should make sure that duplicate laboratory reports, duplicate dictations of hospital records, paid insurance claims, and other extraneous and unnecessary paperwork are eliminated from the file.

Retaining Tax Records (Retention Schedule)

The Internal Revenue Service (IRS) requires that records supporting items of income or deductions in a tax return be retained until expiration of the statute of limitations for that return. The statute of limitations for an income tax return ordinarily expires three years after the return is due to be filed or two years from the date the tax was paid, whichever is later. If an amount of income that should have been reported was not reported, and the amount of income is more than 25 percent of the income shown on the return, the statute of limitations does not expire until six years after the return was filed.

If a taxpayer files a fraudulent return, the IRS has an indefinite period for assessment and collection of the tax evaded. The government cannot wait indefinitely, however, to criminally prosecute a taxpayer. Ordinarily the government has three years from the date of a tax crime to commence prosecution. This time is extended to six years if the tax crime charge involved defrauding the government, willful tax evasion, aiding in the preparation of a fraudulent return, willful failure to pay tax or file a return on time, filing a false return, interfering with the administration of the tax laws, or conspiring to commit tax evasion.

In addition to your tax returns, other records should be retained. A guide for retaining records is shown in Figure 8.

Various local, state, and federal statutes and regulations, as well as specific individual needs should be considered before you establish your record retention program. The Office of the Federal Register publishes the *Guide to Record Retention*. This document provides a reference to which records must be kept, by whom, and for how long. Copies of this book may be obtained from the Superintendent of Documents, United States Government Printing Office, Washington, D.C. 20402 (202-783-3238) (see also Appendix 34).

Keeping Patient Records

The length of time that medical records must be preserved is covered by state and local laws. Most states set a minimum of seven to ten years. Problem cases should be kept indefinitely if there is any threat of legal action. X-ray films and histology slides are usually kept indefinitely.

Inasmuch as minors may file a suit after they reach their majority (eighteen to twenty-one years of age, depending on state law) for acts performed during their childhood, it is necessary to keep a minor's record for an appropriate length of time.

In most states suits may be filed for two years after a minor reaches legal age. You should plan on keeping a minor's records for at least two years after he or she reaches majority, again depending on your state statute of limitations.

Terminating a Patient's Care

When a patient's account has become delinquent and requires the services of a collection agency or action in a small claims court, you may find it necessary to terminate the future care of the patient. It is important that you follow the proper procedure for terminating the patient's care to protect yourself

Accident reports and claims (settled cases)	7 years
Accounts payable ledgers and schedules	7 years
Accounts receivable ledgers and schedules	7 years
Audit reports of accounts	Permanently
Bank reconciliations	1 year
Capital stock and bond records, ledgers, transfer registers, stubs showing issues, record of interest coupons, options	Permanently
Cash books	Permanently
Charts of accounts	Permanently
Checks (cancelled, but see the following exceptions)	7 years
Checks (cancelled for important payments, i.e., taxes, purchases of property, special contracts; checks should be filed with the papers pertaining to the underlying transaction)	Permanently
Contracts and leases (expired)	7 years
Contracts and leases still in effect	Permanently
Correspondence (routine) with patients or vendors	1 year
Correspondence (legal and important matters only)	Permanently
Deeds, mortgages, and bills of sale	Permanently
Depreciation schedules	Permanently
Duplicate deposit slips	1 year
Employee personnel records (after termination)	3 years
Employment applications	3 years
Expense analyses and expense distribution schedules	7 years
Financial statements (end-of-year, other months optional)	Permanently
General and private ledgers (and end-of-year trial balances)	Permanently
Insurance policies (expired)	3 years
Insurance records, current accident reports, claims, policies	Permanently
Internal audit reports (in some situations, longer retention periods may be desirable)	3 years
Inventories of products, materials, and supplies	7 years
Invoices from vendors	7 years
Journals	Permanently

Figure 8. Records retention schedule.

Minute books of directors and stockholders, including bylaws and charter	Permanently
Notes receivable ledgers and schedules	7 years
Option records (expired)	7 years
Payroll records and summaries, including payments to pensioners	7 years
Petty cash vouchers	3 years
Property appraisals by outside appraisers	Permanently
Property records—including costs, depreciation reserves, end-of-year trial balances, depreciation schedules, blueprints, and plans	Permanently
Savings bond registration records of employees	3 years
Stenographer's notebooks	1 year
Stock and bond certificates (cancelled)	1 year
Tax returns and worksheets, revenue agents' reports, and other documents relating to determination of income tax liability	Permanently
Time books	7 years
Trade mark registrations	Permanently
Vouchers for payments to vendors and employees (includes allowances and reimbursement of employees, and officers for travel and entertainment expenses)	7 years

Figure 8. (Continued)

against a lawsuit based on abandonment of the patient.

You should send a letter to the patient by certified mail indicating that you are terminating care. The letter should be addressed and delivered to the patient only. A signed, return receipt from the post office should be requested. The letter to the patient should state that you are terminating care because of lack of payment of the patient's account. You should indicate that your care will terminate at some reasonable period of time in the future, usually within a week from the date of the letter. The letter should also state that in the interim, care will be provided, but only in emergency situations.

The letter should indicate that the patient has the

responsibility for obtaining another physician, and that your office will forward medical records to any physician of the patient's choice upon receipt of proper authorization for release of records. You might also state in your letter that further action, as provided by law, may be taken if the patient's bill remains unpaid. You must be cautious, however, that the letter is not drafted in terms that threaten or harass the patient. The following is a sample letter terminating a patient's care.

Dear Mr. __________,

Your account has remained unpaid since __________. My office staff has made multiple attempts to inform you about your unpaid balance and tried to make arrangements for convenient payments to meet your budget. Your account still remains delinquent.

I therefore find it necessary to inform you that I am terminating your professional care. Since your condition requires medical attention, I suggest that you place yourself under the care of another physician.

I will continue to provide care in the event of an emergency for a reasonable period of time after you have received this letter but in no event for more than one week.

You are responsible for selecting another physician to assume your future care. On receipt of proper authorization from you, I will make available to any physician of your choice your case history and information regarding diagnosis and treatment you received from me.

Most sincerely,

John Smith, M.D.

Prescribing Controlled Substances (Narcotics)

The federal regulations dealing with the prescribing of controlled substances can be found in the United States Code Annotated Title 21, sec. 811 et seq. A printed copy of the complete regulations that implement the Controlled Substances Act of 1970 may be obtained from the Superintendent of Documents, United States Government Printing Office, Washington, D.C. 20402 (202-783-3238). These regulations outline the federal law. However, there are also many state laws that place further restrictions on prescribing controlled substances. You should seek the advice of your attorney regarding both state and federal laws before prescribing such drugs. The federal regulations recognize five schedules of controlled drugs.

1. *Schedule I substances.* This classification includes those drugs that have no accepted medical use in the United States and have a high potential for drug abuse, such as heroin, LSD, peyote, and mescaline.
2. *Schedule II substances.* These drugs have a high potential for drug abuse with a tendency toward severe psychic or physical dependence. Drugs in this schedule include certain narcotics, stimulants, and depressants. Examples of schedule II drugs are hydromorphone (Dilaudid), meperidine (Demerol), oxycodone (Percodan), the amphetamines, phenmetrazine (Preludin), methylphenidate (Ritalin), and the barbiturates.
3. *Schedule III substances.* The drugs included in this schedule all have a potential for abuse, but of a lesser degree than those in schedules I and II. Examples of such drugs are glutethimide (Doriden), methylprylon (Noludar), and paregoric.
4. *Schedule IV substances.* The drugs in this schedule have even less abuse potential than those listed in the previous schedules and include such drugs as ethchlorvynol (Placidyl), meprobamate (Equanil), chlordiazepoxide (Librium), diazepam (Valium), oxazepam (Serax), clorazepate dipotassium (Tranxene), flurazepam (Dalmane), and propoxyphene (Darvon).
5. *Schedule V substances.* These drugs have a minimal potential for drug abuse and consist primarily of compounds containing narcotic drugs for use as antitussives and antidiarrheals.

If you plan to regularly dispense any scheduled medications from your office, you will be required by federal law to keep detailed records and make an inventory every two years of your complete stock of controlled substances. This record must be kept for two years. A copy of it does not have to be submitted to the United States Department of Justice, Drug Enforcement Administration (DEA) unless requested.

If you wish to dispense controlled drugs from schedule II in your office or carry controlled drugs in your medical bag, you must obtain an order form from the DEA to purchase the drugs. The order form must be submitted in triplicate.

A written prescription is required for all drugs listed in schedule II. The prescription must be signed by the physician. A rubber stamp signature will not be accepted by a pharmacist. Refills of prescriptions for schedule II drugs without a new signed prescription are prohibited. Those drugs that appear in schedules III, IV, and V, however, may be prescribed either over the telephone or in writing.

Prescriptions for controlled substances may only be renewed five times within a six-month period from the date of issuance of the initial prescription. A new prescription is then required either orally or in writing from the physician.

Any physician who stores controlled substances in his office must keep the drugs securely locked in a well-constructed cabinet or safe. Theft of controlled substances must be reported at once to the regional DEA agency (see Appendix 18). The local police authorities should also be notified.

The DEA publishes a small physician's manual, which may be ordered at no cost by writing to the United States Department of Justice, Drug Enforcement Administration, Registration Section, Post Office Box 28083, Central Station, Washington, D.C. 20005 (202-633-1249).

Assignments, Authorizations, and Releases

When a patient comes to your office for the first time you may wish to obtain multiple release forms for purposes of providing other doctors and insurance companies with information in the patient's record as well as obtaining information from other doctors (Fig. 9). It may also help you to have an insurance assignment of benefits release form on file in your office. This obviates the need to repeatedly contact your patient to sign additional insurance forms to assign their insurance benefits. It also assists you in the collection of your professional fees in those occasional instances when a patient moves and cannot subsequently be located to sign an insurance release form.

ASSIGNMENTS, AUTHORIZATIONS, AND RELEASES

RELEASE OF INFORMATION

I authorize ________________ (doctor's name) to release to any insurance company or governmental agency (example, Blue Cross/Blue Shield or Medicare) any medical information contained in my records, when such material is required in connection with determining a claim for payment. I authorize ________________ (doctor's name) to release any medical information accumulated in the course of my examination or treatment to any other doctor, hospital, or nursing home. I authorize the release of any medical information contained in any other doctor's or hospital records to ________________ (doctor's name).

INSURANCE ASSIGNMENT

I authorize payment from any insurance company or any governmental agency (example, Blue Cross/Blue Shield, Medicare, etc.) directly to ________________ (doctor's name) for any medical or surgical benefits otherwise payable to me for the services of ________________ (doctor's name) but not to exceed the reasonable and customary charge for these services.

AUTHORIZATION OF CARE AND ACKNOWLEDGMENT OF RESPONSIBILITY FOR PAYMENT

I authorize ________________ (doctor's name) to examine me and make such tests and perform such procedures as are reasonable and necessary in the diagnosis and treatment of my case. I agree to pay ________________ (doctor's name) the professional fees in return for the above rendered services. I agree that should the amount of any insurance benefits be insufficient to cover the professional fees of my care I will be responsible for the payment of the difference. I agree to pay the entire amount of my professional fees if my professional fees are not covered by insurance benefits.

SERVICE CHARGES

I agree to the payment of a reasonable service charge not to exceed $5 per month based on the actual administrative costs of rebilling, if my account is overdue.

ORIGINAL ASSIGNMENTS, AUTHORIZATIONS, AND RELEASES ON FILE

I permit a copy of the above assignments, authorizations, and releases to be used in place of the original, which has been filed in the office of ________________ (doctor's name).

X ________________________________ ________________

Patient's signature Date

Figure 9. Sample authorization for release of information.

You may wish to have your patient agree to the payment of a reasonable service charge if the patient's account becomes overdue. The American Medical Association Judicial Council has ruled that it is not improper for a physician to add a service charge on overdue accounts that have not been paid within a reasonable time; however, the charge must closely approximate the actual administrative cost of rebilling the patient. The patient must be notified in advance of the existence of this practice and the charging of a service charge may require adherence to further disclosure requirements under the Federal Truth in Lending, Consumer Credit Protection Act. You should also obtain a ruling from your county and state medical societies regarding the propriety of making a service charge on overdue accounts before initiating this practice in your office.

After-Hours Pharmacy Calls

You should make it a routine practice to discourage pharmacy calls requesting prescription refills after your office is closed. Refills for prescriptions should be made only during your office hours when your patient's chart is available for you to review.

On weekends and after hours, some physicians authorize pharmacies to give patients enough medication to refill a prescription for a day or two and request that the pharmacy or the patient call their office during office hours to obtain authorization for additional medication. You should make a record of all after-hour prescription refills that you have authorized. This record should be put in the patient's chart for future reference. If you have a call-in dictation system or telephone answering machine in your office, this type of information should be dictated at the time the prescription is refilled.

Lists of Telephone Numbers

Your office aide should keep a list of all your current patients' names, addresses, and telephone numbers. This may take the form of a card file in hanging trays or a file on a rotating wheel (Rolodex type). Either type of index can be easily purged and updated. In addition to a list of your current patients, your file should include all individuals who are called frequently, for example, your broker, accountant, attorney, equipment salespeople, pharmaceutical company representatives, and other business associates. The hanging files and rotary wheel files can be purchased from an office supply company and come in various storage sizes.

In addition to maintaining a file in your office for telephone numbers, it is helpful for you to carry a small pocket notebook that contains a listing of your most frequently called telephone numbers. These numbers might include those of referring physicians, local pharmacies, and business associates. Carrying this notebook can save you substantial time.

Professional Courtesy

The Hippocratic oath says ". . . I will keep this oath and stipulation: To reckon him who teach me this art equally dear to me as my parents, to share my substance with him, and relieve his necessities if required; to regard his offspring as on the same footing with my own brothers . . ." The American Medical Association Code of Ethics proposes that a physician "cheerfully and without recompense give his professional services to physicians or their dependents."

Professional ethics and local custom will dictate your policy regarding professional courtesy. There are a number of patients to whom professional courtesy might be extended. Certainly professional ethics require that you extend professional courtesy to a physician, either active or retired, and his or her immediate family members (spouse and children). You will have to decide whether to extend courtesy to such persons as osteopaths, chiropractors, dentists, dependent parents of doctors, nondependent parents of doctors, registered nurses, licensed practical nurses, hospital employees, employees of other doctors' offices, hospital technicians, teachers, clergy, and pharmacists.

You should prepare a bill for your services for all individuals to whom you extend professional courtesy. It is medically ethical for you to file for any insurance benefits that a recipient of professional courtesy might have. Professional courtesy recipients are often grateful having you file for these fees so that they do not feel guilty not paying for your services. Your receipt of insurance payment also relieves the recipient from the possible burden of trying to reciprocate with a gift or other service.

When You or Your Family Are Recipients of Professional Care

When you or your family receive professional care you should offer to assign any insurance you may have to the physician caring for you. It is a personal choice, but highly recommended that you carry full insurance coverage for both yourself and your family members. Your care or your family's care is thereby not rendered at a loss to the provider of this care. You can feel that no less time or care will be given to you because you are a non-paying patient.

Insurance policies for yourself, your family, and your office staff may be obtained at group rates through numerous medical and dental societies. The premiums are usually inexpensive and frequently tax deductible. If your practice is incorporated, the insurance premiums may be paid for by your corporation under a medical and dental reimbursement plan.

If you are the recipient of professional care that is not totally compensated by insurance you might consider giving your doctor a gift or a donation to a charity in his or her name. This may be given as a Christmas present. Remember that this is a token of thanks—it cannot and should not try to replace dollar for dollar the value of services.

After-Hours Telephone Calls

You should provide your answering service with guidelines for screening telephone calls after your office has closed for the day. You may establish categories into which you wish your answering service to divide your calls. These categories might include routine patient calls, urgent patient calls, emergency patient calls, hospital calls, emergency hospital calls, pharmacy calls, and personal calls.

Instruct your answering service to screen and categorize all of your calls in the best way possible. You should then specify preferences for accepting various categories of calls. For example, some doctors specify that they do not wish to be contacted between 11 P.M. and 7 A.M. about routine patient calls related to appointment cancellations or new appointments.

To minimize the number of interruptions, let your answering service know when you are dining, attending social events, or otherwise engaged, with instructions to hold your calls except for emergencies. Some physicians call their answering services at periodic intervals to pick up groups of calls rather than have the answering service interrupt them each time a call is received.

Every physician establishes a routine for handling telephone calls, but since telephone calls represent the greatest potential for interrupting your personal and professional life, careful planning of a system to handle calls coordinated with your answering service is imperative.

Insurance Claims

Almost all insurance claims filed by your office will fall into one of five major categories.

1. *Blue Cross/Blue Shield.* Blue Cross/Blue Shield is a nonprofit corporation that sells health insurance. Blue Cross provides hospital benefits. Blue Shield covers doctor's fees. Every state has its own Blue Cross/Blue Shield program (see Appendix 16).

   A physician who agrees to participate in the Blue Shield program agrees to provide services to Blue Shield subscribers and accept payment according to Blue Shield regulations. The Blue Shield participating physician participates in two basic Blue Shield contract agreements: the indemnity contract and the usual, customary, and reasonable (UCR) contract.

   Indemnity contracts cover the majority of Blue Shield subscribers and provide a partial payment of physician fees according to a predetermined fee schedule. Blue Shield pays the doctor directly and the doctor may bill the patient for any difference between his or her fee and the indemnity schedule fee.

The second type of Blue Shield agreement is the UCR contract. Whenever a physician provides care for a patient covered by a UCR contract, the physician must accept whatever the Blue Shield program allows as a full fee.

Under the UCR Blue Shield contracts, payments to the physician are based on usual, customary, and reasonable charges. These are defined as follows:

a. *Usual*. The fee usually charged by an individual physician to a patient (i.e., his or her own usual fee).
b. *Customary*. That fee within the range of fees usually charged by physicians of similar training and experience for the same service in the same geographic area; the so-called community fee.
c. *Reasonable*. The fee determined by a medical review panel where circumstances of a case are unusual.

The Blue Shield carrier determines the usual fee and the customary fee on a percentile method. A decision is made to accept a certain percentile as the one most equitable to all concerned (physicians and patients). For example, the federal Medicare program uses the 75th percentile for customary or community fees and the 50th percentile for usual fees when establishing guidelines for reimbursement payments.

After determining an acceptable percentile, all of a physician's fees for a specified service and a specific time period are assembled in the order of lowest to highest charges. The same process is followed to determine the lowest to highest charges for the same specific service and time period for all physicians within the geographic area with similar training and experience.

The determination of the maximum fee to be paid by the Blue Shield carrier is then made by finding the fee from the predetermined percentile of usual fees, and similarly, the fee from the predetermined percentile of customary fees. If there is a difference between the usual and customary fee, the Blue Shield carrier allows the payment of the lower of the two fees.

Consider the following example. During a single year Dr. Smith submits charges ranging from $300 to $375 for performing an appendectomy (his usual fee). After analyzing his range of charges and the number of times each charge was made, the Blue Shield insurance carrier can calculate his 90th percentile charge. Assume his 90th percentile charge amounts to $365.

During the same year all of the surgeons in Dr. Smith's area submitted their charges for an appendectomy in amounts ranging from $200 to $395. Assume that the 90th percentile charge for all the surgeons amounts to $350 (the customary or community fee).

In this example, Blue Shield will pay up to $350 for Dr. Smith's appendectomy fee, representing the lesser of the 90th percentile of Dr. Smith's usual fee ($365) and the 90th percentile of the community or customary fee ($350).

You should write to your state Blue Shield office to obtain the *Blue Shield Manual for Physicians.* This manual contains all of the information about the Blue Shield program needed for filing claims.

2. *Medicare.* Medicare is a federal health insurance program for people over the age of sixty-five and for those people severely disabled under the age of sixty-five who are eligible. The Medicare program is designed to help pay part of their health care costs.

   There are two parts to Medicare: part A, hospital insurance, and part B, medical insurance. Part A, the health insurance portion, helps pay for inpatient hospitalization and for certain followup care after the patient leaves the hospital. Part B, the medical insurance portion of the program, helps pay for the doctor's services, outpatient hospital services, and other medical items and services not covered by the hospital insurance portion of the program.

Medicare Part B medical insurance funding comes jointly from those who sign up for Part B benefits and from the federal government. The insurance premiums are automatically deducted from monthly benefit checks for those who request Part B coverage and receive Social Security benefits, railroad retirement benefits, and civil service annuities. Others who are not Social Security recipients and who qualify for Medicare benefits must pay premiums directly to the Social Security Administration. The federal government pays about two thirds of the premium costs for medical insurance, and the Medicare recipient pays approximately one third of the total premium cost. Medicare Part B provides the following benefits:

a. Payment of 80 percent of the reasonable medical charges made by a doctor. The *reasonable medical charge* is the amount that the Medicare intermediary considers a fair charge for the procedure. The Medicare intermediary arrives at the reasonable medical charge in the same way Blue Shield reimbursement fees are determined. The patient is responsible for the remaining 20 percent of the reasonable medical charges and also for a yearly deductible of seventy-five dollars (in 1982).
b. Outpatient hospital visits are covered subject to the same 20 percent co-insurance and seventy-five-dollar yearly deductible.
c. One hundred home visits made by allied health professionals, such as speech therapists and physical therapists, are payable at 100 percent of cost after the deductible has been met.

Medicare Part B benefits are available to pay a doctor's fees on an *accept assignment* basis or on a *not accept assignment* basis. If the doctor agrees to accept assignment, Medicare pays the doctor 80 percent of the reasonable charges after the patient's seventy-five-dollar deductible has been met. The payment goes directly to the doctor. The doctor may bill the patient, but only for the 20 percent co-insurance and any unpaid balance of the deductible that was withheld from the doctor's payment.

If a doctor or a patient submits a claim to Medicare for payment of professional fees on a not accept assignment basis, the payment is made directly to the patient and the patient is responsible for paying the total doctor's fee regardless of amount. For a patient to submit a claim he or she must fill out the Medicare form, SSA–1490, attach the doctor's bill, and submit the form to the Medicare intermediary. Some doctor's offices complete this form as a service for their patients. For a patient to submit his or her own claim, the doctor's office must provide a signed and itemized statement of services rendered.

The following example shows the differences between the two types of assignment for a theoretical medical bill of $150.

Accept Assignment		*Not Accept Assignment*	
Medicare reasonable medical charges	$125	Medicare reasonable medical charges	$125
Medicare pays 80%	100	Medicare pays 80%	100
Patient is billed for 20% co-insurance	25	Patient is billed	150
Doctor receives check directly from Medicare	100	Patient receives check directly from Medicare	100
Doctor writes off	25	Doctor writes off	00

Certain charges are not covered by the Medicare program. A few such non-covered charges include:

Routine physical examinations
Routine foot care
Eye examination for prescribing eyeglasses
Ear examinations for prescribing hearing aids
Cosmetic surgery
Immunizations or injections unless required because of injury, infection, or treatment of disease states
Drugs with or without a prescription

If Medicare does not pay for a service, the patient is responsible for paying for the service whether the physician accepts assignment or does not accept assignment. Medicare and Blue Shield follow the same policy in paying the physician either the prevailing (customary or community) fee or the physician's usual fee, whichever is lower.

On July 1 each year the Medicare intermediary updates each physician's fee profile of usual charges for the previous year, and makes a cost-of-living adjustment for the Medicare prevailing charges (customary or community fee).

The Freedom of Information Act permits you to receive a copy of the Medicare prevailing charge fee profile and your own usual charge profile by making a written request to your Medicare intermediary for this information.

3. *CHAMPUS*. CHAMPUS is an abbreviation for Civilian Health and Medical Program of the Uniform Services. It is a program that provides health benefits for dependents of active military personnel, retired military personnel, and their families. Under the CHAMPUS program, qualified recipients who go to a civilian physician for medical care have a portion of the physician's fees paid for by the federal program. CHAMPUS benefits are roughly equal to those for the Medicare program. The intermediaries that administer the CHAMPUS program are listed in Appendix 23.
4. *Third-party insurance programs*. Filing claims with an insurance company for professional fees has been simplified by the introduction of uniform health insurance claim forms (see Your Initial Printing Requirements, p. 32). In April of 1975, the American Medical Association approved the uniform claim form for use with group and individual insurance claims. This form has not, however, been completely accepted by all third-party insurance carriers, and its acceptance varies from locality to locality. Many Blue Shield plans accept the uniform health insurance claim form, but it is suggested that you contact your area representative to find out local policy. At present CHAMPUS has accepted the uniform health insurance claim form in only a few areas of the country. Almost all general insurance carriers do accept it. The uniform health insurance claim form may be ordered from the American Medical

Association or from a medical printing company (see Appendix 24).

A special form of third-party insurance payment is Workers' Compensation. Workers' Compensation covers medical expenses and disability benefits for workers whose injuries or illnesses are the result of their jobs. All employers with more than a specific number of workers as established by state statute are required to carry Workers' Compensation insurance. The employer may write an insurance contract through an insurance carrier of his or her choice. A special claim form is designated by the state, and claims are filed with the insurance carrier. The state establishes the allowable fee schedule for medical services and the physician is paid directly by the insurance carrier. The medical and surgical fee schedule and up-to-date information about Workers' Compensation programs may be obtained from your state's Director of Workers' Compensation (see Appendix 22).

5. *Medicaid.* The Medicaid program is a medical program established to assist the needy. It is administered jointly by the federal and state governments. Each state operates its own program based on guidelines established by the federal government. Medicaid benefits cover private physician fees, hospital charges, and certain drug expenses. An individual must show proof of poverty before qualifying for Medicaid benefits. He or she must earn less than a specific minimum yearly salary and have no significant assets. The individual may be the beneficiary of another insurance program, but any other insurance proceeds collected must be subtracted from any Medicaid benefits paid and refunded to the Medicaid program.

   The doctor's fees are paid by the program administrator directly to the physician. The fees paid by the Medicaid program are generally less than those paid by Medicare and private insurance carriers for similar services.

   If you accept a Medicaid patient and file for his or her Medicaid benefits as payment of your professional fees, you are obligated by law to accept this amount as payment in full. You may not bill the patient for any additional fees not covered by the Medicaid program.

It is because of this poor funding policy and the overwhelming multiplicity of social and economic problems that many physicians avoid accepting Medicaid patients.

Submitting Insurance

At the time that your office aide submits a patient's insurance claim form requesting that insurance benefits be sent to your office for payment of the patient's professional fees (assignment accepted), you should send the patient a copy of his or her itemized bill with a notation that you have submitted the bill and insurance forms to the insurance carrier. You should also make a notation to the patient that if there is any remaining balance after the insurance company has paid its benefits, the patient will be billed for the difference. A copy of an itemized bill with the aforementioned notation should be rubber stamped *Not Sufficient for Insurance*. The physician's signature should not appear on this copy of the bill. By stamping the bill in this way you safeguard against the occasional dishonest patient who files a copy of the itemized bill carrying the doctor's signature and receives payment directly from the insurance carrier, then subsequently refuses to pay your professional fees, pocketing the insurance check.

Treatment of Minors

If your practice involves the care of infants, children, or minors, you should familiarize yourself with the state statutes regarding the rights of minors and the responsibility of parents. In general, parents are liable for the care of their minor children. In all cases try to inform parents as to what your treatment program will be (see also Informed Consent, p. 121). Even if the parent is not present there is good legal precedent that parents must provide for the care of their children, and are therefore responsible for your fees. If there is any question regarding the initiation of care for a minor child, be sure to consult your attorney.

If you care for the minor children of divorced parents, be sure to find out which parent is legally responsible for the child's medical support. The fact that a parent has custody of a child does not necessarily mean that he or she is legally responsible for payment of medical fees. Be sure to have your office aide establish who is responsible for the bill when registering a new minor child.

Patient Education

Patients expect and have the right to a clear explanation of their medical problems and recommended therapy. You must continually strive to communicate this information to your patient on a level that the patient can understand. The recent vogue of patients requesting second opinions from other physicians is probably not so much an outgrowth of the consumer movement to control medical costs and curb unnecessary medical and surgical procedures as it is a failure by physicians to clearly communicate their impressions to patients and their families.

Patient education is a form of communication designed to make the patient knowledgeable about normal human physiology and the pathophysiology of disease states. The time taken by the physician to educate patients about their disease processes ultimately results in time saved for the physician. Patients who are knowledgeable about their illnesses have a tendency to call their physicians less often. Family members who are knowledgeable about their relative's illness take less of the physician's time inquiring about the patient's illness and progress. Patients and families have less anxiety related to illness when the physician has attempted to educate them. Furthermore, the risks of medical malpractice actions are substantially reduced if physicians clearly communicate with patients and their families.

There are numerous educational techniques that can be used in your office and hospitals. Although no technique is a substitute for direct communication with the patient by the physician, there are many aids that act as an extension of your voice.

1. *Patient education by your office personnel.* One of your office aides may be given the responsibility to expand and elaborate on your explanations, instructions, or advice; for example, dietary instructions given to diabetics, preparations for special x-rays, or care of wounds and dressings.
2. *Books and pamphlets.* Many well-written, scientifically accurate pieces of literature are available in handout form for the patient's education. Pharmaceutical companies usually distribute these booklets free of charge (see Pharmaceutical Company Representatives, p. 62). Patients appreciate reading material concerning their illness and its treatment. Consider writing your own educational booklet about a particular medical topic if you treat the illness according to your own unique modes of therapy or if satisfactory general literature is not available.

   The Pharmaceutical Manufacturers Association, 1155 Fifteenth Street, NW, Washington, D.C. 20005 (202-463-2000), produces a catalog of films and publications that is useful for patient educational purposes. There is no charge for printed materials, and films are loaned subject to payment of return postage.
3. *Models and charts.* Patients have a better understanding of human illness if explanations can be supplemented with demonstrations on models and charts. Scientific supply companies and some pharmaceutical companies have plastic models of various organ systems available, such as accurate, anatomically constructed models of the heart, lungs, digestive system, and brain (see Appendix 33). Graphic illustrations of organ anatomy and pathology are also available in the form of booklets and wall charts. All of these forms of visual communication help your patient understand his or her illness and your proposed therapy.
4. *Audiovisual aids.* Several companies have developed audiocassettes dealing with common disease entities and medical conditions. The cassette can be played for patients in the office on an in-

expensive tape recorder. In 1982 a satisfactory cassette tape recorder could be purchased for less than fifty dollars. Examples of such instructional cassettes include a series sponsored by the Milner-Fenwick Company with topics such as hypertension, diabetes, and peptic ulcer disease (see also Appendix 33). For those disease entities that you treat commonly and discuss frequently with your patients, you should consider making your own tape recordings discussing the pathophysiology and your approach to therapy. You might also consider making similar cassette recordings for those medical and surgical procedures that you commonly perform, outlining the nature of the procedure, the indications for the procedure, and the potential risks and complications associated with the procedure. Although your recorded cassette is not a substitute for your own personal explanation about a particular illness or procedure, it can complement and amplify your explanation and serve as a means of obtaining informed consent (see Informed Consent, p. 121).

More elaborate audiovisual education systems have been devised combining the audiocassettes with projected slide images illustrating the information as it is presented on the cassette tapes. Several companies manufacture and distribute the equipment needed for presenting this educational material (see Appendix 36). Some hospitals offer patient education programming over a closed-circuit television. You should ask the head of the hospital's professional relations department or director of medical education whether your hospital has a closed-circuit television system. You may be able to televise your own patient education material explaining and illustrating your medical and surgical procedures for replay through the hospital television system.

Other sources available for obtaining audiovisual materials for patient education include

National Audio-Visual Center
General Services Administration
Washington, DC 20409
301-763-1872

National Archives Trust Fund Board
National Archives Building
Washington, DC 20408
202-523-3170

Public Health Service Audio-Visual Facility
Center for Disease Control
1600 Cliston Road
Atlanta GA 30303
404-329-3311

By adopting these and other forms of educational communication you will save time, allay patient anxiety, reduce medical–legal risks, and promote the growth of a successful practice.

5. Hospital Patient Management

Time for Rounding

Consider having your office hours or surgical schedule at times that differ from the traditional rounding and operating room schedules. Internists and family practitioners traditionally round in the early morning and see office patients throughout the remainder of the day. Surgeons generally round early in the morning, operate in the morning, and then see patients in their offices in the afternoon.

When you round during morning hours patients are frequently in the x-ray department, taking their baths, eating breakfast, having physical therapy, or otherwise indisposed. In addition, the patient's x-ray and laboratory results are not usually available until later in the afternoon. You may also find that there is competition early in the morning among nurses, attending physicians, and consultants for the patient's chart. For all of these reasons you should consider changing your schedule to use time slots that are not used by others.

The internist might consider seeing office patients early in the day and round in the middle or late afternoon. This work pattern also makes it possible to see new patients who have checked into the hospital that day during afternoon rounds. It also eliminates the need to return to the hospital a second time, which would be necessary in the case of a traditional morning rounding schedule.

A surgeon may find that operating room time is easier to schedule in the afternoon. Surgeons who switch to the use of afternoon operating time may find it necessary to convince their associates to adopt a similar rounding and operating room schedule to assist each other in the operating room.

Informed Consent

A physician has a duty to adequately inform the patient before initiating treatment. This is known as obtaining *informed consent*. Obtaining informed consent must be done with the idea of countering potential claims by the patient that (1) the patient did not recall being told of the risks of treatment, (2) the patient did not recall signing the consent form, and (3) the patient did not realize what he or she was signing. Effective consent includes a discussion of the following:

What is to be done
Why the treatment or procedure is necessary or desirable
What alternatives are available
What risks are associated with the proposed treatment
By whom the treatment or procedure is to be performed

How much you must inform a patient about a procedure, operation, or treatment may vary from jurisdiction to jurisdiction. A number of jurisdictions adhere to the rule that disclosure of risks is governed by the custom of other physicians in the community. The Supreme Court of Arizona stated in the case of Riedisser v. Nelson, 534 P.2d 1052 (Ariz. 1975), ". . . the duty of disclosure of the risks by the physician or surgeon is measured by the usual practices of the medical profession."

A slightly different viewpoint has been taken in some jurisdictions holding that the physician's duty to inform is measured by what a hypothetical reasonable physician would disclose under similar circumstances. This viewpoint was expressed in the case of William v. Meneham 379 P.2d 292 (Kans. 1963):

> . . . it is the duty of a doctor to make a reasonable disclosure to his patient of the nature and probable consequences of the suggested or recommended treatment, and to make a reasonable disclosure of the dangers within his knowledge which are incident or possible in the treatment he proposes to administer. But this does not mean that the doctor is under obligation to describe in detail all of the possible consequences of treatment. . . . The duty of the physician to disclose is limited to those disclosures which a reasonable medical practitioner would make under the same or similar circumstances.

However, the trend has recently been to measure the physician's duty to disclose by the patient's "need to know." In these cases the patient's right to decide can be exercised only if the patient has sufficient information to make an intelligent choice. The physician's duty is no longer measured by community medical practice standards nor by what a hypothetical "reasonable physician" would tell the patient. A physician's duty to disclose potential risks is judged by whether the information presented or omitted by the physician in the disclosure is material to an intelligent decision by the patient. These cases have dramatically altered the doctrine of informed consent by making the patient's point of view, not the physician's, the controlling factor in determining whether consent was truly informed. (See Canterbury v. Spence, 464 F.2d 722 [D.C. Cir. 1972], and Cobbs v. Grant, 502 P.2d 1 [Cal. 1971].)

The following suggestions are made to help you obtain adequate informed consent:

1. Make sure your consent form gives specific details relating to the recommended procedure or treatment. The consent form should include possible complications and the likelihood of a complication occurring.
2. Avoid using a consent form that is so lengthy that a patient cannot read or understand it.
3. Avoid the use of complex medical terminology in your consent form.
4. Personally explain to the patient and, if possible, family members, any proposed procedure or treatment including potential risks and complications. This responsibility cannot be delegated to a nurse, receptionist, or other paramedical aide. Only the physician can be expected to answer all of the patient's questions related to the proposed procedure or treatment. It is therefore the physician's duty to personally inform the patient regarding the proposed procedure or treatment.
5. Have the signing of your consent form witnessed by a family member as well as one of the nursing staff, paramedical personnel, or your office staff. The exact time and date of the signatures should be recorded on the consent form.
6. Have the consent form signed in your presence. This act allows you, the physician, to personally verify that the risks and alternatives of treatment were explained to the patient; that the

patient was given ample opportunity to ask further questions; that the patient understood the potential risks of the proposed procedure or treatment; and that the patient or responsible family member signed the consent form.

7. If possible, make sure that the patient was not under the influence of narcotics, sedatives, or tranquilizers when the proposed treatment or procedure was explained and when the consent form was signed.
8. Consider using attention-getting devices in your consent form if there is any concern that the patient's comprehension of the consent form or of your discussion is incomplete. For example, have the patient fill in blank spaces on the form or read and initial each paragraph of the consent form.
9. Make special efforts to educate your patient about proposed procedures and treatments. Some physicians prepare their own information sheets or booklets about procedures and treatments. Other physicians prepare tape recordings explaining their most common procedures or operations. Some physicians use videotapes played over the hospital's closed-circuit television system as an educational tool to help obtain informed consent (see also Patient Education, p. 117). The information sheets, booklets, and recordings should not serve as a substitute for your personal discussion with the patient and the patient's family regarding the proposed procedure or treatment.
10. After each discussion with a patient about a proposed procedure or treatment, make a note in the hospital chart or your office records that the proposed procedure or treatment was discussed. Include in your note that you discussed potential risks and complications listing several examples. State in your note that the patient appeared to understand the explanation of the proposed treatment or procedure and its associated risks; and having no further questions the patient was willing to proceed.

Obtaining informed consent from incompetent patients presents special problems. Incompetent patients include children and adults who cannot consent owing to mental or physical disability.

Minors. The general rule is that the parent or legal guardian of a minor must give consent for a surgical procedure or other medical treatment. You should first ascertain the legal age of majority in the state in which you practice. The age of majority is eighteen in all but six states. In Alabama, Nebraska, and Wyoming the age of majority is nineteen. In Kentucky, Mississippi, and Missouri the age of majority is twenty-one (although minors over the age of 18 in Missouri and over the age of 14 in Alabama may consent to their own medical care).

Many states have adopted specific statutes allowing minors to consent to certain procedures before they reach their age of majority. Examples include donating blood and receiving treatment for venereal disease and alcohol or drug abuse. The United States Supreme Court has also upheld the right of minors to obtain abortions without parental consent.

Most states allow minors to consent to treatment if they are (1) emancipated, (2) have been or are married, (3) have had a child, (4) have served in the armed services, or (5) have graduated from high school. Emancipated minors are generally defined as minors no longer requiring the support of their parents as evidenced by one or more of the following: (1) they are living apart from parents, (2) they are financially independent, and (3) they are free from parental control or discipline. Some states have adopted the "mature minor" rule that allows minors to consent to treatment as determined by their comprehension of the nature and consequences of the treatment without regard to age.

Incapacitated adults. Adults that cannot give consent on their own behalf must have consent given for them by another person before treatment can be initiated. Every state has a legal procedure for declaring a person incompetent. Some states have statutes that specifically delineate who may consent for an incompetent patient if no official guardian has been designated. It is common practice for physicians to seek consent from a patient's spouse, next of kin, or others who have been providing for the patient when no official guardian has been appointed. This practice may be acceptable unless a

Surgical Consent Form

1. I, ______________, authorize Dr. ______________, associates, and such assistants as may be selected to treat the following condition(s):
   ____
   (description of the condition and need for treatment)
   ____
   ____
2. Dr. ______________ has explained the procedure required to treat my condition, and I understand it to be as follows:
   ____
   (description of the procedure or treatment in lay terms)
   ____
   ____
3. I understand that during the course of the operation, unforeseen conditions may become apparent that require an extension of the original procedure, or a different procedure from that described above. I therefore authorize Dr. ______________, associates, or assistants to perform the surgical procedure that they, in the exercise of their professional judgment, feel is necessary and desirable. This authority [ ] shall [ ] shall not (check one) extend to the treatment of conditions requiring treatment that are not known to my physician at the time the operation is begun.
4. Dr. ______________ has explained to me that the following risks and possible consequences are associated with this procedure:
   ____
   (to be completed by the physician)
   ____
   ____
   ____
5. Dr. ______________ has informed me of the following alternatives to the procedure:
   ____
   ____
   ____

Figure 10. Surgical consent form.

controversy over the intended treatment arises, in which case the physician should request that a court order be obtained to declare the patient incompetent and to appoint an official guardian.

You should ask your attorney to review the consent forms that you use for all procedures and treatments. Legal advice regarding consent is particularly important in certain special situations including

Sterilization
Termination of life-support measures
Abortions

6. I authorize the hospital to dispose of tissue, organs, or body parts in accordance with its usual policies.
7. I have been informed that there are risks inherent in the performance of any surgical procedure including severe loss of blood requiring blood transfusions, infections, blood clots going to the lungs, and cardiac arrest. I am aware that the practice of medicine and surgery is not an exact science and acknowledge that no guarantees have been made to me about the results of the operation or procedure.

____________________ ____________________
(Witness) (Patient's signature*)

____________________ A.M. P.M.
(Date) (Time)

* Because the above patient is an unemancipated minor, _____ years old, or is unable to sign for the following reasons:

____

____

the above consent is given for the patient by:

____________________ ____________________
(Witness) (Closest relative or legal guardian)

____________________ A.M. P.M. ____________________
(Date) (Time) (Relationship)

I have personally explained to ____________________ the nature of
(Patient or representative)

the patient's condition, the proposed procedure or treatment, and the risks involved, as described in 1, 2, and 4 on

____________________ at ____________________ A.M. P.M.
(Date) (Time)

____________________ ____________________
(Witness) (Physician's signature)

____________________ A.M. P.M.
(Date) (Time)

Figure 10. (Continued)

Medical examinations following sexual assault
Modification of standard treatment because of a patient's religious convictions
Blood tests for police purposes

See Figure 10 for a sample surgical consent form.

Keeping Track of Your Hospital Patients

Every doctor with a hospital practice must develop a system to keep track of his or her hospital census. The development of this system is basically a communication between you and your office staff. This communication should include the name of the patient in the hospital, the room number of the patient in the hospital, and the type of service performed on the patient. There are a number of systems that can be used successfully.

1. *Index card or note system.* Some physicians mark the name and room number of the patient on a three- by five-inch index card and make a daily notation for each service performed. Such a card might look something like this.

   Patient name: John Doe
   Room number: 24
   September 17, 1980—initial hospital care, history, and physical examination—$60
   September 18, 1980—interpretation of electrocardiogram—$20
   September 18, 1980—routine hospital visit—$15
   September 19, 1980—critical care unit visit—$30

   The same entries can be made on small notebook paper and carried in a loose-leaf, pocket-sized notebook. When the patient leaves the hospital, the notebook paper or the index card can be handed in to your business office. Since your office staff should have a formalized fee schedule, you may not need to include fee entries on your daily notation cards unless the fee varies for some reason from your usual charge. When you turn in your cards or notebook slips for billing, you may also make notations to your billing clerk regarding special handling of the account, such as

   a. Bill insurance only
   b. Accept Medicare assignment
   c. Do not accept Medicare assignment
   d. Bill patient directly—patient has no insurance
   e. No professional charges—patient is indigent
   f. Professional courtesy

   The index card or notebook system is best adopted by an internist or family practitioner who may have patients in the hospital for extended periods of time, and who are charging fees daily for hospital visits and other professional services.
2. *The daily list system.* A second system for keep-

ing track of your patients in the hospital is the daily list system. Each day your front office prepares a list of names and room numbers of patients that you have in the hospital. If you are asked to see additional patients in consultation during the day, you may add the new names to your list. Each morning you turn in your old list to your secretary with billing information. Your office aide prepares an updated list for the next day.

The advantage of the daily list system is that this regular communication between you and your office aides permits them to keep you up-to-date on such additional information as meetings, appointments, or new patients coming into the hospital, as well as surgery or procedures scheduled that day. The daily list system adapts well to the surgical specialist, who may have as many patients to see as a family practitioner or an internist, but charges an all-inclusive fee for a surgical procedure without regard to follow-up visits.

Discharging Patients

When you discharge patients from the hospital, allow yourself additional time to spend with the family and the patient. It is certainly ethical and legitimate to charge a slightly higher fee for this prolonged visit. It is worth your time to reduce further questions and post-discharge telephone calls by outlining for the family and the patient the four Ds.

1. *Diagnosis.* Be explicit about your impression of the patient's problem. You may wish to review the laboratory findings, films, electrocardiograms, and other objective findings with the patient and his or her family. At this time you can also check the record thoroughly before discharging the patient so that you do not overlook a possible abnormal test result. It is always best to catch these abnormalities while the patient is still in the hospital than to catch them at the time you dictate your final discharge summary after the patient is

at home. It is better still to have these abnormal results reviewed and corrective action taken before your chart is returned to you from the hospital audit committee.

2. *Diet.* Tell the patient what kind of diet to follow after being discharged from the hospital. Most patients insist on some form of dietary instruction. If the patient's diet is unrestricted make this clear to both patient and family at the time of discharge. Plan to have the dietician see the patient and the family several days before discharge if a special diet is to be prescribed. At the time of discharge reemphasize the dietary instructions and refer to the dietician's literature.
3. *Drugs.* Write your prescriptions and get into the habit of asking the pharmacy to label the contents of each drug bottle. When writing the prescription, give the patient some idea of what the drug is prescribed for, for example, "Valium, 2 mg as needed for anxiety." Be sure to caution patients—and record that you have cautioned them in your discharge note—about any potential major side effects the drug may cause. By recording this information, you minimize potential medical-legal problems.
4. *Disposition.* Tell the patient when to return to your office for follow-up care or when to return to the office of the referring physician. If possible, leave an order for the ward secretary to schedule the follow-up appointment, and give the patient a written appointment reminder before the patient leaves the hospital.

Your final discharge visit should also include instructions to the patient as to the allowable level of activity. You should cover such things as when the patient can return to work, when the patient can resume driving an automobile, and how much physical activity to resume over the days and weeks after discharge from the hospital. You may find it appropriate to discuss resumption of normal sexual activities. Patients who have had babies, gynecologic and urologic surgery, cardiovascular surgery, myocardial infarcts, as well as other serious operations, illnesses, or injuries may be concerned about this issue but be embarrassed or reluctant to talk about sexual matters. Consider including advice on these matters as part of your routine predischarge counseling.

After you instruct the patient and family on the four Ds and post-discharge activity level, this information should be recorded in outline form as your final discharge progress note. This outline will be a helpful guide when you dictate your final discharge summary.

Dictation of Your Discharge Summary

All hospitals require the completion of a final discharge summary after the patient has been discharged. There is certain basic information that should be included in the summary. Remember that the document is a *summary* and does not have to enumerate every detail related to the patient's hospital stay. For many physicians, the preparation of a discharge summary is a chore with low priority. The presentation of a concise discharge summary, however, can be a learning experience for the physician preparing the summary, a potential teaching tool for a referring physician, and a source of information for subsequent treatment or readmission of the patient to the hospital. In addition, the summary can demonstrate your sense of organization, showing other physicians your ability to care for patients referred to you.

At the end of your discharge summary, you should give instructions to the transcriber to prepare extra copies for the referring physician, consultants, and possibly for the patient, if these are your wishes. The following information should be included in your discharge summary:

1. Name of the patient
2. Hospital number
3. Date of admission
4. Date of discharge
5. Referring physician, if any
6. A concise statement of clinical data, which need not repeat the complete history and physical examination, but should include

   a. The reason for the patient's admission to the hospital
   b. A simple statement referring the reader to the admitting history and physical examination

7. Names of consultants
8. Hospital complications (e.g., wound infections, shock, pulmonary emboli)
9. Surgical and special procedures performed
10. Laboratory data
11. A concise summary of the hospital course including major happenings during the patient's hospital stay
12. Final discharge diagnoses, subcategorized into the patient's primary diagnoses or active problems and the patient's secondary diagnoses or inactive problems
13. Discharge diet
14. Discharge drugs
15. Discharge disposition, including a statement about the patient's discharge activity, ability to return to work, and follow-up laboratory testing
16. Discharge disability, including a statement that the patient has
    a. No disability on leaving the hospital
    b. Temporary disability for a defined period of time
    c. Possibly total, permanent disability
17. The patient's condition at the time of discharge, which might be described as one of the following:
    a. Ambulatory
    b. Improved
    c. Able to care for his or her daily needs
    d. Mentally able to attend to his or her administrative affairs

6. *Financial Management*

Pegboard Accounting

1. *Purpose of the pegboard system.* There are numerous ways to keep track of your daily charges. One of the most convenient is the *pegboard system,* so designated because a rigid board with pegs on the left-hand margin holds the transaction forms. Forms with carbon and corresponding holes are placed over the pegs. By using the pegboard system your office aides make one writing step and complete the following three transactions:

   a. A record of the transaction on your daily log of charges and receipts
   b. An update of the patient's account receivable card
   c. A receipt and record for the patient of that day's charges, also serving as the patient's reminder of the next appointment and as a record for the patient to use for filing an insurance claim

2. *Operation of the pegboard system.* Your office aide follows five steps to operate the pegboard system.

   a. At the beginning of each day's transactions a log sheet of charges is placed on the pegboard. A group of prenumbered, preshingled charge slips is pegged into position over the log sheet (Fig. 11).
   b. When the patient is seen for an appointment, his or her account receivable card is pulled from the file. The patient's balance is then entered on the right-hand side of the charge slip. This entry is simultaneously recorded on the log sheet, since the account receivable card is pretreated with a no-carbon-required chemical. The record on the log sheet represents the patient's previous balance.
   c. The right-hand portion of the charge slip containing information about the patient's previous balance is detached along the perforation on the slip and placed in the patient's

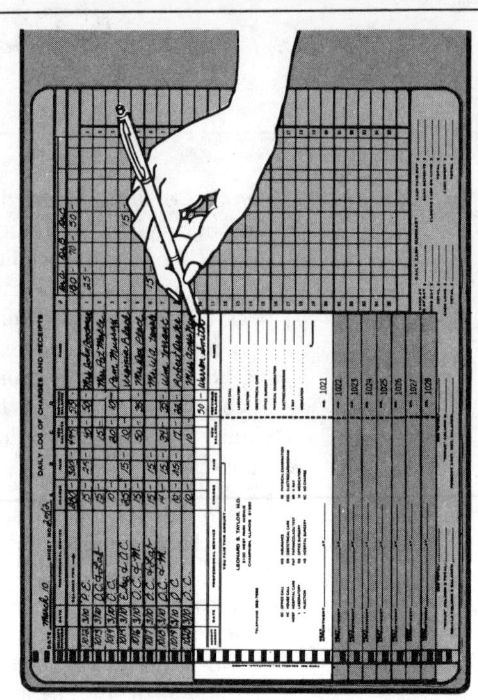

B

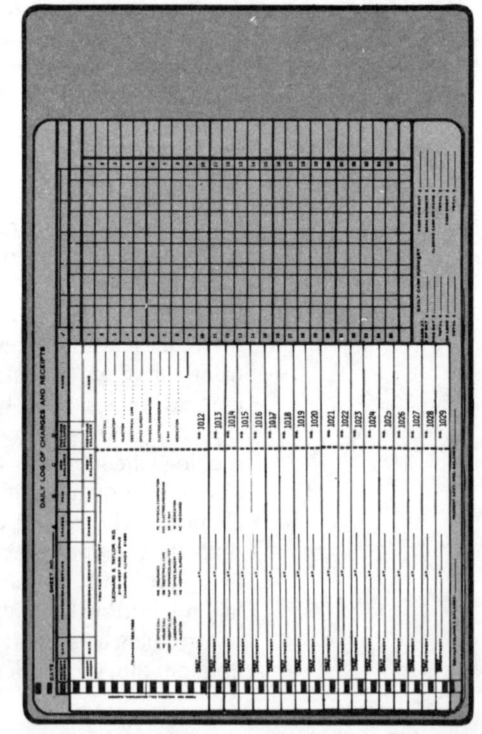

A

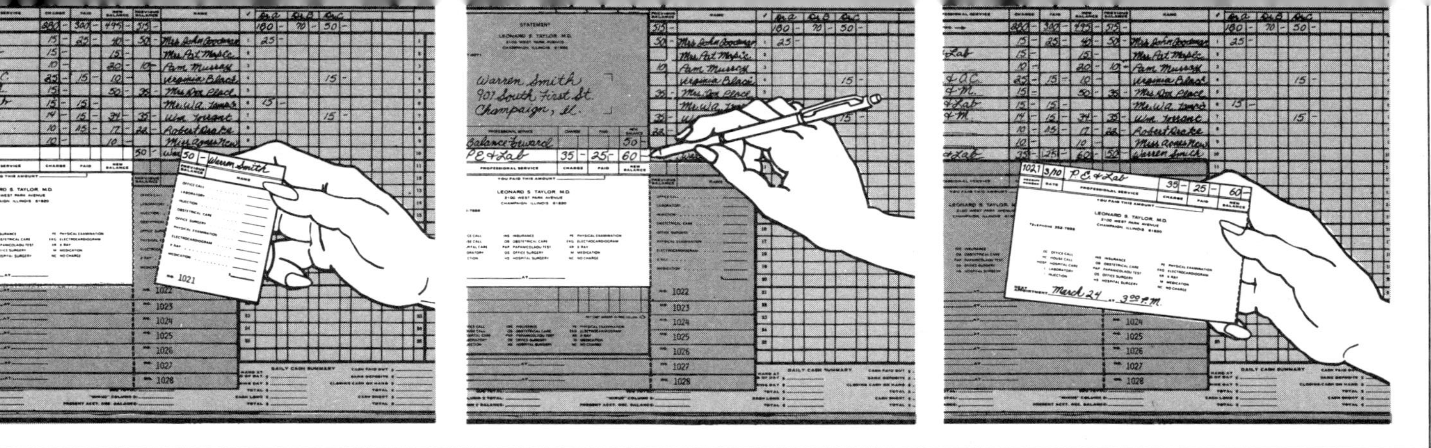

Figure 11. The pegboard system. A. To begin, a daily log of charges and receipts is placed on the pegboard. A set of imprinted, prenumbered, and preshingled receipt and charge slips is then pegged into position so that the top posting line of the top receipt slip is directly over the first open posting line on the daily log sheet. B. When the patient arrives, his account record or account receivable card is pulled from the file. The patient's name is entered on the first available charge slip, along with the receipt number and any prior balance shown on the account receivable card. One writing automatically records this information in the proper column on the daily log sheet. C. The charge slip is detached along the perforated line and forwarded to the doctor along with the patient's chart. When treatment is complete, the doctor fills out the charge slip and gives it to the patient to return to the business desk. D. When the charge slip is returned to the business desk, the patient's account receivable card is positioned under the correct receipt form. The date, services rendered, charge, payment (if any), and new balance due are then posted in one step on the account receivable card and daily log sheet E. The receipt slip is removed from the pegboard and handed to the patient. This gives the patient the option of sending in payment before the costly step of a month-end statement becomes necessary. The date and time of the patient's next appointment, if applicable, may be noted in the space provided on the receipt slip. Additional columns are provided on the day sheet to show distribution of charges or receipts among two or more partners, or for departmental income records. Figures can be noted in these columns after the patient leaves. (Courtesy of the Colwell Company, Champaign, IL.)

medical file. The file and attached charge slip are then forwarded to the doctor. The doctor is thereby made aware of the current status of the patient's account balance. The remaining left-hand portion of the charge slip stays attached to the pegboard until the patient leaves the office. On completion of the patient's examination, the doctor notes the fees on the detached portion of the charge slip that has accompanied the patient's record and gives it to the patient to return to the front office. This gives the patient a chance to see the status of the account and the fee for current service. Seeing the bill tends to encourage in-office payment.

d. When the charge slip arrives at the front office, the patient's account receivable card is again placed under the correct prenumbered left-hand portion of the charge slip that remained attached to the pegboard. The account receivable card is lined up to the charge slip. A single entry is made on the charge slip for the date, services rendered, charges, payment, and new balance due. These same entries are simultaneously recorded on the account receivable card and the log of charges.
e. The charge slip is then removed from the pegboard and given to the patient. Space may be provided at the bottom of the charge slip for scheduling the patient's next office appointment.

3. *The superbill system.* There are numerous variations on the pegboard system, one of which is known as the *superbill.* The superbill charge slip also serves as an attachment to an insurance claim form to expedite preparation of an insurance claim. The superbill charge slip usually contains the standard procedural code numbers to meet Medicare, Blue Shield, and third-party insurance carriers' standards. With the superbill, you can prepare in a single step a charge slip for the patient that simultaneously serves as a portion of an insurance claim form, with no additional time spent by your office personnel filling out insurance forms (Fig. 12).

ELISABETH J. ANDERSON, M.D.
Family Practice
1900 OAKHILL BOULEVARD, SUITE 84
HEAVENLY VALLEY, CALIFORNIA 96979

CAL. LIC. # A-1111
SOC. SEC. # 000-11-2222
PROVIDER # OOA555566Z

TELEPHONE: (987) 654-3210

☐PRIVATE ☐BLUE CROSS ☐BLUE SHIELD ☐IND. ☐MEDI-CAL ☐MEDICARE ☐OTHER:

PATIENT INFORMATION

PATIENT'S LAST NAME FIRST INITIAL	BIRTHDATE / /	SEX [ ] MALE [ ] FEMALE	TODAY'S DATE / /
ADDRESS CITY STATE ZIP	RELATIONSHIP TO SUBSCRIBER	SOCIAL SECURITY NUMBER	
SUBSCRIBER OR POLICYHOLDER	INSURANCE CARRIER		
ADDRESS CITY STATE ZIP	INS. ID	COVERAGE CODE	GROUP
OTHER HEALTH COVERAGE? – [ ] NO [ ] YES – IDENTIFY	DISABILITY RELATED TO: [ ] Accident [ ] Pregnancy [ ] Ind. [ ]	DATE SYMPTOMS APPEARED, INCEPTION OF PREGNANCY, OR ACCIDENT OCCURRED: / /	
ASSIGNMENT: I assign & request payment of medical benefits to undersigned physician for services described below. SIGNED: (Patient or Parent if Minor) Date:	RELEASE: I hereby authorize undersigned physician to furnish information to my insurance carriers concerning this illness or accident. SIGNED: (Patient or Parent if Minor) Date:		

✓	DESCRIPTION	CODE/M.	FEE	✓	DESCRIPTION	CODE/M.	FEE	✓	DESCRIPTION	CODE/M.	FEE	✓	DESCRIPTION	CODE/M.	FEE
	1. OFFICE VISIT – NEW PATIENT				4. OFFICE SURGERY				5. INJECTIONS				9. HOSPITAL SERVICES		
	Limited	90010			Post-Op	90050			Interm. Jt./Bursa	20605			Admit: / / Dsch: / /		
	Intermediate	90015			Biopsy	27045			Major Jt./Bursa	20610			Surgery Date: / /		
	Comprehensive	90020			Excision/Biopsy	27045			Tendon Sheath	20550			[ ] Hosp. Visits @ $ ea.		
					Burn Care	16000			Therapeutic Inj.	90730			Dates:		
	2. OFFICE VISIT – EST. PATIENT								Therapeutic Inj.	86585					
	Brief - Triple Rx	90040			Cystoscope	52000			Tine Test	86585			Admit - H & PE	90220	
	Limited	90050			Coleman Dil.				Turbinate	30200			Hospital Visit	90250	
	Intermediate	90060			Excise Lesion:								CCU/ICU Visit	90296	
	Extended	90070			Benign	114							Discharge	90275	
	Comprehensive	90080			Malignant	116			6. LABORATORY						
	Comp.- Complex	90085			F.B. Removal:				Gram Stain	87205					
	By Report	90086			Cornea	65220			Sed. Rate	85650			Surgical Assist	-80	
	Annual Physical	90088			Conjunctival	65205			Urinalysis	81000					
					Tissue	10120			Wet Mount	87210					
	3. OFFICE PROCEDURES				I & D				Pap Smear	88100			Dr.:		
	Anoscopy	40260			I & D - Seb. Cyst	10003							10. CONVALESCENT HOSPITAL		
	Audiometry	92551			I & D - Abscess	10060			7. CAST & SPLINTS				Initial-Intermed.	90318	
	Ear Irrigat. (1-5)	69210			Inject. Bursa/Jt.	20550			Short Arm Cast	29075			Limited-new ill.	90351	
	EKG	93201			Lumpectomy	19120			Long Arm Cast	29065			Limited-same ill.	90352	
	EKG w/Interp.	93203			Repair, Intermed.	120			Short Arm Splint	29125			Intermediate	90361	
	Fluroscope	76000			Repair, Complex	131			Long Arm Splint	29105					
					Repair: Scalp, Neck, Etc.				Short Leg Cast	29425			11. CLERICAL		
	Joint Aspiration	206			To 2.5 cm	12001			Short Leg Splint	29515			Insurance Billing	500	
	Nail Avulsion	11730			2.5 to 5.0 cm	12002			Removal	29700			Medical Reports	99080	
	Nail Debridement	11700			Repair: Face, Ears, Etc.								Written Reports	501	
	Nail Matrix	11750			To 2.5 cm	12011									
	Proctosigmoid	40240			2.5 to 5.0 cm	12013			8. SUPPLIES	99070			12. MISCELLANEOUS		
	Spirometry	94600			Vasectomy	55250			Ace Bandage Arm Sling						
	Tonometry	92100			Wart Removal	17110			Dressing Sterile Tray						
									Finger Spl. Plaster Spl.						
									Plaster Cast Gelo Cast						

DIAGNOSIS:

SERVICES PERFORMED AT:
[ ] Office [ ] St. Columba's Hospital [ ] General Hospital [ ]
[ ] E.R. 109 Rosemount Lane 4400 West Main Street
[ ] Pleasant Valley, CA 96966 Heavenly Valley, CA. 96979

DATES DISABLED:
FROM: / / TO: / /
OK TO RETURN TO WORK: / /

RETURN APPOINTMENT INFORMATION:
5 · 10 · 15 · 20 · 30 · 45 · 60
DAYS WKS. MOS. PRN

NEXT APPOINTMENT:
M – T – W – TH – F – S
DATE: / / TIME: AM PM

DOCTOR'S SIGNATURE/DATE

ACCEPT ASSIGNMENT? [ ] YES [ ] NO

INSTRUCTIONS TO PATIENT FOR FILING INSURANCE CLAIMS:

1. COMPLETE UPPER PORTION OF THIS FORM.
2. SIGN & DATE.
3. MAIL THIS FORM DIRECTLY TO YOUR INSURANCE COMPANY. YOU MAY ATTACH YOUR OWN INSURANCE COMPANY'S FORM IF YOU WISH, ALTHOUGH IT IS NOT NECESSARY.

REC'D. BY:
[ ] CASH
[ ] CHECK
[ ]

TOTAL TODAY'S FEE	
OLD BALANCE	
TOTAL	
AMT. REC'D. TODAY	
NEW BALANCE	

INSUR-A-BILL ® • BIBBERO SYSTEMS, INC. • SAN FRANCISCO • © 8/81

Figure 12. "Superbill" claim form. The claim form is detached from the pegboard and sent into the treatment area along with the patient's chart. At the end of the visit, the doctor completes the treatment portion of the form. Entering necessary data is easy and accurate because the form can be preprinted with the most frequently used procedure codes for your practice. The claim form is then handed to the patient for return to the business desk. (Courtesy of Bibbero Systems, Inc., San Francisco.)

4. *Materials needed for the pegboard system.* To purchase a basic pegboard system, you will need the following:

   a. Pegboard
   b. Ledger card tray to hold your accounts receivable cards
   c. Alphabetical index guide for the accounts receivable cards
   d. Log sheets for charges and receipts
   e. Accounts receivable cards that are chemically pretreated so that no carbon paper is required
   f. Charge slips custom designed to represent the most common types of services performed in your office.

   The price of a system containing 200 log sheets, 500 accounts receivable cards, and 1,000 charge slips was approximately $150 in 1982. The expense may be greater depending on the size and complexity of the charge slips and the quantity of forms ordered. There are a number of companies that sell complete business office financial systems including the pegboard system. It is generally more expensive to buy a system from companies, such as Control-o-fax, Safeguard, and McBee, that offer complete financial systems than it is to buy from a printing company. However, most business system companies offer the services of a business representative who will train your office personnel in the use of a pegboard system and offer to develop a total business system in your office to cover such things as check writing, billing and collection systems, payroll disbursements, and cash control systems. A number of medical printing companies have duplicated the franchised business system components and sell them directly to customers (see Appendix 24).

Balanced Books

Your accountant will help you set up your accounting books when you go into practice. One of your aides with a head for figures and a knack for using a calculator can be instructed to do daily bookkeeping chores. A trained bookkeeper is not absolutely necessary and represents a luxury that the physician starting practice usually cannot afford.

Your accountant will help your office aide establish a cash receipt journal. The journal will show the total amount of funds received in the office each day. You will also require a disbursement journal to record an itemized list of amounts paid for such things as rent, salaries, Social Security taxes, drugs, supplies, laboratory fees, car expenses, postage, telephone expenses, laundry, interest payments, and taxes. It is from these journals that your accountant will be able to prepare your taxes and produce a balance sheet showing your assets and liabilities.

How to Avoid Embezzlement

The key to avoiding embezzlement in your practice is to establish good financial controls. Good financial controls include the following:

1. Physician involvement in the business aspects of the practice

    a. Only the doctor should have the authority to sign checks. The role of writing checks may be delegated to an office aide, but all checks should be signed by the doctor. Avoid using signature stamps.
    b. The doctor should review all invoices before signing a check for payment.
    c. A small fund of cash should be established to make change for patients. This fund should be separate from your petty cash fund and should be balanced on a daily basis (see also Cash in the Office, p. 143).
    d. The doctor should periodically open all mail. This act confirms your interest in the business aspect of the practice and provides an internal spot-check for letters from patients who may complain that their account balances have not been properly credited. Repeated complaints by patients about bookkeeping errors may be a clue that an employee is embezzling funds.

e. The doctor should review the patient's account receivable card and check the patient's credit balance before signing a refund check to a patient.

f. Only the doctor should authorize writing off a patient's balance. The doctor should initial the account receivable card of any patient whose account balance is written off. An employee should not be given the authority to write off a patient's account balance. Allowing an employee to write off a patient's account balance provides the employee with the opportunity to embezzle payments made by a patient.

g. The doctor should periodically spot-check the daily log of charges and payments (daysheet), the ledger cards, and the charge tickets for any unauthorized alterations.

h. The doctor should review all cancelled checks returned by the bank at the end of the month. The doctor should have the envelope containing the bank statement and cancelled checks left unopened on his or her desk. This act prevents a dishonest employee from removing cancelled checks that have been altered. The doctor should consider having the bank statement and cancelled checks sent directly to his or her accountant.

2. Accounting systems and internal controls

   a. If possible, have different members of your office staff be responsible for the handling and recording of financial transactions. For example, the office aide who opens the mail might not be the aide who records and totals the daily log of charges and payments; or the aide who records and totals the daily log of charges and payments might not be the aide who totals and prepares the daily bank deposit. Also consider rotating among office aides the responsibility for handling and recording financial transactions.

   b. Insist that the daily log of charges and receipts be balanced at the end of each day.

   c. Record all billing charges and cash receipts promptly.

d. At least once a month—and preferably more often—have one of your office aides add up all the ledger card account balances. Make sure the total balance matches the cumulative total of your accounts receivable control on your log of charges and receipts. The most common discrepancy will be that the ledger card balance is less than the daysheet accounts receivable control balance. This discrepancy generally occurs because an office aide did not have possession of all ledger cards when the balance was tabulated. The ledger cards may have been misplaced in the patient's file folder, left with your insurance clerk, or be in the hands of an office aide working on delinquent accounts. To avoid misplaced ledger cards and reduce the discrepancy between the ledger card total and the accounts receivable control total, make sure that an "out card" listing the name of the patient, the patient's current balance, and the location of the account receivable card is left in the tray of ledger cards whenever a ledger card is removed from the ledger card tray. Have your office aide prepare the ledger card balance on an adding machine or calculator that produces a tape. The tape will help your office aide find any errors in addition as well as transcription errors.
e. Have all of your office charge tickets numbered consecutively. Make sure that all charge tickets are accounted for at the end of each day. The charge tickets should never be destroyed. Your office aide should void all charge tickets that might otherwise be destroyed, and retain the charge ticket in a permanent binder in its consecutive number sequence with all your other charge tickets.
f. Establish an *audit trail* from the appointment book to the log of charges and receipts, and from the record of receipts to the bank deposit. Make sure that all patients who make and keep their appointments and are seen in your office have a recorded entry on your log of charges, even if no charge is made (e.g., a postoperative follow-up visit). Periodically

spot-check to make sure your patient appointments coincide with the entry of patients seen on your daily log of charges. Insist that every patient appointment—even work-ins—be logged in your appointment book, and likewise on your copy of the daily schedule of office appointments to be seen. Make sure that all receipts of cash and checks can be reconciled with your daily bank deposit slip.

g. Consider bonding all of your employees (see Buying Insurance, p. 147).

Keeping Tax Records Organized

You should provide your accountant with an accurate and detailed account of all your professional expenses. This account is your best guarantee for going through an Internal Revenue Service (IRS) audit without penalties.

You should record *all* of your income for services paid by patients no matter how it is received. Whether you get paid in cash on a house call, by check in the office, or by payment in the mail, be sure that your office staff credits the payment to the patient's account and deposits the payment. Remember that the patient will be listing his or her payment as a medical deduction for income tax purposes at the end of the year, and that these deductions may be compared with your records by the IRS.

To provide a record of your transportation expenses you should use a credit card with a major oil company, MasterCard, or VISA. A majority of these expenses may be deductible, but only with adequate records. If you select one of the major credit cards for charging transportation expenses and other office expenditures, do not use the same charge card for personal expenditures. Obtain a second major credit card for personal use. This system automatically helps you separate expenses incurred on a professional basis from charges incurred on a personal basis. Use the major credit card that you have selected for charging professional expenses when entertaining professionally. Be sure you document on the charge ticket the name of the guests and the professional nature of the entertainment for audit purposes.

Your best protection against IRS audit is the maintenance of accurate, detailed, and validated records. Your daily record-keeping habits will help your accountant meet tax deadlines without disturbing you at inopportune times because he or she needs information to complete your records.

The IRS provides a free guide with useful tax information for persons starting small businesses. You may write to the Department of the Treasury and request Publication 333 (revised November 1980), *Tax Guide for Small Business.* The government also provides a toll-free telephone number in each state to call for answers to your federal tax questions (see Appendix 26).

You should also keep a copy of the IRS Tax Calender in your office so that your financial secretary may refer to it. The tax calender is revised and published each year. It may be obtained free of charge from your local IRS office.

Another useful guide that should be obtained is *Your Business Tax Kit.* The IRS has assembled this kit and will provide it free of charge. It will help you comply with federal tax laws and regulations. Request Publication 454 (revised July, 1980).

Cash in the Office

Do not keep a large petty cash fund in your office. Twenty-five to fifty dollars in cash is adequate. This money should be kept in small bills and change. Keeping larger amounts of cash in the office invites theft. The petty cash fund should be used primarily to pay for spur-of-the-moment expenses and small items. All other items of office expenses should be paid for by check.

To establish your petty cash fund, write a check payable to "cash," labeling it "for petty cash." As money is paid out of the petty cash fund, receipts are left for each expenditure. Before writing another check to replenish the petty cash fund, you should review the receipts, make sure the receipts total the sum of the allocated petty cash fund, and then staple the receipts to the original check used to draw the money for the fund. The receipts will provide a record of payment for your accountant.

The petty cash fund should be kept separate from the small amount of cash kept in your office with which to make change for patients paying their fees with large-denomination bills. You should never allow a patient to cash a personal check and receive payment from the change fund or from the petty cash fund. Do not allow patients to overpay their bills for professional fees and receive change from the change fund or from the petty cash fund.

Payments received in the office should be deposited on a daily basis regardless of the amount. Your office aides should not keep payments overnight in your office. Deposit slips should be kept on file to compare and validate your daily accounting sheets with the end-of-the-month bank statement (see also How to Avoid Embezzlement, p. 139).

A word about safety: Let your office employees take the daily deposit to the bank during daylight hours. If your employee must take the deposit after hours, the deposit should be sent to the bank in a locked deposit bag, which the bank will provide for your office. The deposit should be placed in the bank's night depository.

Receiving a Worthless Check

When a patient's check for professional fees is returned to your office because the patient has insufficient funds in his or her bank account, you should take the following steps:

1. Return the check to the patient's bank and ask the bank to hold the check until the patient deposits additional funds.
2. Notify the patient that the check has been returned for insufficient funds. Most states have laws dealing with the issuance of worthless checks. Most state laws require the holder of the check to notify the person who issues the check that it has been dishonored and give the person a specific number of days from receipt of notice to pay the check in full plus a defined service

charge. Notification should be made by certified or registered mail. The person receiving the certified or registered notification should be required to sign a return mail receipt provided by the post office for a small additional fee. This receipt serves as proof of notification. If the issuer of the check does not pay the check in full, including the service charge, many state laws allow for criminal prosecution. You should consult your attorney regarding your legal right to recover fees in these circumstances.

Every patient who writes a check in your office to pay professional fees should have identifying information recorded on the back of the check. Such information might include the patient's full name, address, home telephone number, business telephone number, place of employment, sex, date of birth, height, weight, race, driver's license number, and credit card information. Having this information is essential for identifying and tracing the patient who has passed a worthless check. Most of this information can be obtained from the patient's registration or history form filled out during the initial office visit, and can be supplemented by information on his or her driver's license. Office supply companies can prepare a rubber stamp with spaces to fill in the above information, to be used by your office aides.

Credit Card Charging for Professional Fees

The American Medical Association has approved the use of credit cards for patients paying their professional fees. However, you should obtain the approval of your county medical society ethics committee before establishing a credit card program for your patients. In the last few years, an increasing number of professionals, including doctors, dentists, and attorneys, have started to accept credit card payments for professional fees. Two of the leaders in the credit card industry, VISA and MasterCard, have credit plans that can be introduced into a doctor's office. A local bank usually sponsors the combined VISA and MasterCard credit plans. The bank provides the doctor's office with all the necessary charge tickets, imprinting machines, and identification signs and materials. Patients may charge their professional fees—usually up to a specific dollar limit (in some cases $250)—without the need for the office aide to call the central credit computer for authorization. The signed charge tickets are the equivalent of cash and are deposited into a checking account that the doctor must maintain at the same bank that sponsors the credit card program. The bank makes a charge for the credit card service. The charge is negotiable and depends frequently on the estimated credit risk of the clients and the monthly dollar amount of fees charged. The charge for a credit card program is usually in the range of 2½ to 5½ percent.

1. *Advantages of a credit card program.* The advantages of offering a credit card program to your patients include

   a. Convenience for your patients
   b. Improved cash flow for the doctor's office since immediate payment is received
   c. Reduced problems for the doctor's office with collecting overdue or bad accounts, with the responsibility for debt collections transferred to the bank sponsoring the VISA and MasterCard program

2. *Disadvantages of a credit card program.* Some disadvantages of offering a credit card program to your patients include

   a. Possible reduction of your professional image to the level of a general merchant
   b. Reduction of the amount you collect of your professional fees by the amount of the bank's credit card service charge from patients who have charged their professional fees. Most of the patients who have the economic means to qualify for credit cards usually have the economic means to pay their bills in full
   c. Possible service charge by the bank sponsoring the program if no credit transactions take place during any one month

Buying Insurance

When you go into practice, you will need various types of insurance. You should buy this insurance as a knowledgeable consumer. The proper types of contracts should be purchased and skillfully arranged by you and your insurance representative into a program designed to fulfill your needs. The reason to obtain any insurance is to cover a potential risk to your health or property. The following are a few of the types of insurance you should consider buying.

1. *Life insurance*. Life insurance can accomplish two objectives. The first is to guarantee the existence of a fund of money to pay your final expenses including tax liabilities and provide a source of income for your dependents if you as a breadwinner should die prematurely. The second is to save a fund of money as part of your own living assets for future needs. The first objective is for protection; the second for savings. There are three basic types of life insurance policies.

   a. *Term insurance*. Term insurance is solely for financial protection in the case of death. Term insurance has the lowest premium price. It does not have any cash surrender or loan value.
   b. *Whole life (ordinary life)*. Whole life insurance with its multiple variations is a combination of both a death protection policy and a savings account. Whole life insurance usually has a level premium throughout the life of the insured. Most policies have guaranteed cash values and loan values.
   c. *Endowment or annuity*. Endowment or annuity policies are primarily savings accounts with only small emphasis on death protection. The face amount of the policy is usually payable at the end of a specified contract period or at the time the policy holder dies, whichever occurs first. Annuity contracts allow for various payment options at the time the annuity is paid.

In general, until your income increases, you should consider purchasing maximum term insurance protection and use other types of investments such as stocks, bonds, money market funds, and certificates of deposit for the savings portion of your investment program. There are, of course, exceptions to this plan, which may be pointed out by your attorney, accountant, or insurance representative. You should review your insurance plan annually with your insurance representative, accountant, and attorney. As your income and assets increase, as you grow closer to retirement, and as your dependents become fewer, your needs to cover risks and provide savings through the aforementioned types of insurance will change.

How much insurance you will need when you go into practice will depend entirely on your personal circumstances. If you are thirty years old, married, and have two young, dependent children, you will need more insurance to provide for the needs of your dependents in the event of your premature death than if you are thirty years old, and single (Fig. 13).

You should ask your insurance representative to shop around for the best available rate of life insurance. Premiums vary tremendously from company to company. For example, term policies with equal face values may be offered by one company with an annual premium twice the amount of that of another company. Many professional organizations and state medical societies offer group policies with significant reductions in premiums. Tables 1 and 2 show representative premiums for yearly renewable term and decreasing term life insurance.

2. *Health insurance*. There are four basic types of health insurance benefits that may be purchased in separate contracts or in different combinations.

   a. *Hospitalization*. This contract is intended to pay the insured for hospital expenses including room and board, nursing care, laboratory fees, operating room charges, medicines, and supplies. Try to avoid the purchase of contracts that provide a fixed room rate. Try to obtain a policy that covers the reasonable and customary charges for a semiprivate room.

b. *Medical-surgical reimbursement contracts.* This insurance contract sets allowances for different surgical procedures and medical fees. As with the hospitalization contracts, avoid insurance contracts that specify fixed dollar limits, and seek contracts based on reasonable and customary fees. Although you and your family will receive professional courtesy, you may feel more comfortable buying a medical-surgical reimbursement contract, thereby knowing that medical services from your colleagues will be reimbursed at least to the extent of your insurance coverage.

c. *Major medical insurance.* The major medical contract is designed to meet large medical fees. The contracts are usually issued subject to varying deductible and co-insurance specifications. For example, a major medical policy might have a $100,000 limit for any one accident or illness with a $500 deductible and require 20 percent co-insurance on the first $10,000 of expenses. With such a policy the insured would be responsible for the first $500 of expenses and $2,000 of the next $10,000 of expenses with the insurance company paying for all other expenses up to a maximum of $100,000. There are many combinations of dollar amounts, deductibles, and co-insurances available with varying premiums. You should consider the purchase of major medical insurance coverage with high or no maximum limits to cover the cost of a catastrophic illness or injury.

d. *Disability income insurance.* This insurance contract provides payment when the insured is unable to work as the result of illness or accident. Next to premature death, the greatest economic drain and hardship on your family would be your prolonged disability because of accident or illness. Disability income insurance will cover this risk. This type of insurance should be obtained by a physician as

YOUR FAMILY'S ESTIMATED ANNUAL LIVING EXPENSES	$______
Factors involved in the calculation of this figure will include 1. The age of surviving children and remaining period of childhood financial dependency 2. The age of surviving spouse and likelihood of remarriage 3. The capability of spouse or other surviving family members to gain compensable employment to meet all or part of annual living expenses	
FUNDS REQUIRED TO PROVIDE ESTIMATED ANNUAL LIVING EXPENSES	$______
The size of the fund will depend on 1. The anticipated annual percent yield 2. Whether income generated will be paid from interest only or will be paid out of principal and interest and for what period of time	
FUNDS REQUIRED FOR CHILDREN'S FUTURE EDUCATION	$______
The size of the fund needed to finance children's future education depends on 1. The age and number of surviving children 2. Anticipated educational requirements 3. Estimated inflation factors 4. Anticipated percent return on funds invested	
FUNDS REQUIRED FOR IMMEDIATE PAYMENT OF OUTSTANDING DEBTS	
Office mortgage	$______
Home mortgage	$______
Loans	$______
Estate taxes	$______
Other taxes	$______
Expenses of final illness	$______
Burial expenses	$______
Other expenses	$______
TOTAL FUNDS REQUIRED **(Subtotal A)**	$______
LESS	
ANNUAL SOCIAL SECURITY SURVIVOR BENEFITS	$______
Factors involved in determining survivors benefits include 1. Age of dependent children 2. Number of quarters the deceased contributed toward Social Security benefits 3. Total dollar amount the deceased contributed toward Social Security benefits	

Figure 13. How to estimate life insurance needs.

ANNUAL PENSION PLAN BENEFITS, IF ANY $________

ANNUAL YIELD FROM LIQUIDATED SAVINGS, INVESTMENTS, AND OTHER ASSETS $________

The yield on liquidated assets depends on

1. Anticipated percent yield
2. Whether the income generated is to be paid from interest only or is to be paid out of the principal and interest and for what period of time

EXISTING LIFE INSURANCE $________

TOTAL FUNDS AVAILABLE **(Subtotal B)** $________

TOTAL FUNDS REQUIRED **(Subtotal A)** $________

MINUS TOTAL FUNDS AVAILABLE **(Subtotal B)** $________

LIFE INSURANCE REQUIRED $________

EXAMPLE

John Doe, M.D., age 34, is married with two children ages 6 and 12. John Doe wishes to provide an annual income of $30,000 to cover estimated annual living expenses for his surviving wife and children.

Funds required to provide estimated annual living expenses	$300,000
Funds required for children's future education	25,000
Funds required for immediate payment of outstanding debts	
Office mortgage	–0–
Home mortgage	75,000
Equipment and automobile loans	62,000
Estate and other taxes	10,000
Expenses of final illness and burial	13,000
TOTAL FUNDS REQUIRED **(Subtotal A)**	485,000
LESS	
Annual Social Security survivor benefits	2,000
Annual pension plan benefits	–0–
Annual yield from liquidated savings	8,000
Existing life insurance	25,000
TOTAL FUNDS AVAILABLE **(Subtotal B)**	35,000
TOTAL FUNDS REQUIRED **(Subtotal A)**	$485,000
MINUS TOTAL FUNDS AVAILABLE **(Subtotal B)**	$ 35,000
LIFE INSURANCE REQUIRED	$450,000

Figure 13. (Continued)

Table 1. Representative 1982 Annual Premiums for $500,000 of Yearly Renewable Term Life Insurance

Age	Premium
30	$ 465
35	475
40	575
45	770
50	1,015
55	1,540

Note: The death benefit of a yearly renewable term life insurance contract remains the same throughout the life of the policy. Premium examples are based on nonsmoking males. Premiums are not guaranteed and may vary from company to company and from time to time.

Source: Reproduced with permission of Transamerica Occidental Life Insurance Company, Los Angeles, California.

Table 2. Representative 1982 Annual Premiums for $500,000 of Decreasing Term Life Insurance

Age	15 Year	20 Year	25 Year	30 Year
30	$ 910	$ 920	$1,035	$1,130
35	1,135	1,245	1,435	1,560
40	1,565	1,825	2,125	2,350
45	2,360	2,760	3,180	3,620
50	3,635	4,200	5,245	—

Note: The premium for decreasing term life insurance remains constant throughout the life of the policy. The death benefit decreases monthly over the life of the policy. Currently published premiums are not guaranteed and may vary from company to company and from time to time.

Source: Reproduced with permission of Fidelity and Guaranty Life Insurance Company, Baltimore, Maryland.

soon as possible, even during his or her years as an intern or resident. The cost of the insurance will be based on a number of factors including

(1) Your age at the time the contract is purchased
(2) Your sex
(3) The amount of weekly or monthly dis-

ability income desired (insurance companies will only sell certain limited amounts of coverage based on your current earning capacity)

(4) The waiting period before the benefits are paid: i.e., the shorter the waiting period, the more expensive the policy

(5) Cost-of-living riders which automatically increase the insurance benefit each year based on adjusted cost of living increases without raising the premium

(6) The number of years of disability payments covered by the policy

(7) Whether benefits are payable for non-occupational disability or cover both occupational and nonoccupational illnesses and injuries

(8) Whether recurrent or partial disability is covered

Many state and local medical societies as well as other professional organizations sponsor health insurance policies. Group policies generally have the least expensive premiums, but they can be cancelled if the underwriter cancels the coverage of the entire group. You might consider buying a separate individual non-cancellable policy for a portion of your coverage and a group policy for the remainder of your coverage.

One of the fringe benefits of incorporating your practice is the development of a medical reimbursement plan. The premiums for hospitalization, medical-surgical reimbursement contracts, major medical insurance, and disability income insurance may be paid for by the corporation. The premium is a deductible expense for the corporation and a benefit to you, the employee (see Incorporating Your Practice, p. 165).

3. *Fire and extended coverage.* If you own your office, you will need a fire insurance contract on your building and on the personal property contents within it. Likewise, you will require fire insurance if you own your home. When you obtain a mortgage on your property, either home

or office, the lending institution will require that you purchase some insurance against fire loss.

The basic fire policy covers only fire and lightning. You should purchase an extended coverage endorsement on your basic policy for both home and office to cover such perils as wind storms, hail, explosion, civil commotion, water damage, glass breakage, and fallen trees. These perils are usually subject to a dollar-defined deductible.

The insurance industry now offers comprehensive protection policies combining fire and extended peril coverage for homes that are known as *homeowner's policies*. The same type of comprehensive protection policy may be obtained for business properties as well, covering perils to the building and personal property within the building.

4. *Consequential loss insurance contracts*. These contracts are usually written as endorsements on your office or home fire and extended coverage policies. Examples include

    a. *Business interruption insurance*. This insurance attempts to reimburse the insured for profits and charges lost as a result of damage to property. Usually there must be physical damage to the property requiring total or partial discontinuance of your practice. An important option to consider is payroll endorsement to provide salary payments to your office employees if your practice is interrupted.
    b. *Additional living insurance*. This insurance is designed for a homeowner who must pay normal living expenses when displaced from his or her home because of fire or other insured peril. The same type of rider can be purchased with an office-homeowner policy.
    c. *Accounts receivable insurance*. This insurance pays the insured for losses resulting from inability to collect accounts receivable owing to destruction of accounts receivable records. The insured usually must report the value of the accounts receivable each month. An audit of your accounts receivable at the end of the year helps to determine the actual premium. These insurance contracts may require you to

store your accounts receivable in a safe when your office is closed.

5. *Personal insurance on floating property (floaters).* These insurance contracts reimburse for the theft of personal property. The personal property floater may be written to cover a variety of personal property items. These items need not be listed separately; they are covered by a blanket policy. A personal articles floater is written to cover only specific items of specific dollar amounts and is usually required for fine jewelry, furs, fine art works, stamp and coin collections, silverware, and other personal valuables.

6. *Liability insurance contracts*

   a. *Workers' Compensation insurance.* As an employer you may be required to pay for Workers' Compensation insurance. The laws regulating Workers' Compensation insurance vary from state to state. You should write to your state's regulatory agency to receive information regarding your state's requirements (see Appendix 22).
   b. *Business liability insurance.* A comprehensive general liability policy allows the insured to combine a number of liability coverages in one contract. These coverages include ownership liability in the normal use of your office premises. An endorsement may be added to the basic policy covering medical payments for injuries caused by accidents on the premises. A wide variety of other options can be added to these policies.
   c. *Professional liability insurance.* General liability policies exclude claims for errors committed by a professional in performing his or her duties. Contracts that cover the risks of these errors are commonly referred to as *professional liability* or *malpractice insurance.* Professional liability insurance protects you from claims arising out of alleged malpractice. Practicing medicine without professional liability insurance makes you personally liable to pay damages, court costs, attorneys fees,

and other related expenses if the suit is decided in favor of the plaintiff. A court award of several hundred thousand dollars might result in bankruptcy and the loss of all of your personal assets. Even if you are not guilty of malpractice, the cost of defense and the loss of earnings may be considerable. For all of the above reasons, it is strongly advised that you buy professional liability insurance.

The cost of professional liability insurance may be a major expenditure in your initial practice budget. In most states the premiums are high and physicians in high risk specialties in which the number of claims is greatest may pay from $10,000 to $20,000 per year for coverage.

Your state and county medical societies can advise you about professional liability insurance carriers in your state and can offer guidance about the kinds and amounts of professional liability insurance you should purchase. The amount of professional liability insurance that you will need will depend on your medical specialty, the claims consciousness of your patients, the economic level of your community, and many other factors.

With awards and settlements running into hundreds of thousands of dollars, the trend has been for physicians to buy policies with higher limits. It is not unusual for a physician to carry professional liability insurance coverage with limits from one to five million dollars to protect against large awards and settlements.

d. *Personal liability insurance.* This insurance contract is intended to cover your legal liability arising from maintenance of your home and nonbusiness liability away from your residence. Most insurance coverage for a person's nonbusiness-related liability arising out of negligence is written in a so-called comprehensive personal liability policy. This policy is an all risk policy with few exclusions. The contract usually covers liability for property damage and bodily injury, and in many instances has an option for writing a medical payment rider. As a professional earning a high income, you should consider purchasing a personal liability insurance contract with high contract limits.

7. *Automobile insurance.* When you enter private practice, you should review your automobile insurance coverage and update the limits of coverage. There are five basic parts to your automobile insurance contract.

   a. *Liability insurance.* The liability section of your insurance contract provides you with defense of a suit arising out of the ownership, maintenance, or use of owned and nonowned automobiles. The contract provides payment for bodily injury or property damage arising from a claim against the insured. The contract usually insures members of the insured's household as well as anyone driving the owned automobile with the insured's permission. As with your personal liability insurance contract, your business or office liability insurance contract, and your professional liability (malpractice) insurance contract, you should try to obtain the maximum limits of coverage that are available.
   b. *Medical payments.* Medical payment insurance is designed to pay medical claims of occupants riding in your automobile. Medical payment insurance is usually written with limits of liability per person injured with a maximum limit per accident.
   c. *Uninsured motorist protection.* This form of insurance protection provides coverage for you if you are struck and injured by a negligent motorist who has no liability insurance. Coverage is limited to bodily injury liability claims.
   d. *Physical damage insurance.* This form of insurance provides payments to the insured for damage to his or her automobile for almost any type of peril, regardless of fault. Physical damage coverage includes

(1) Comprehensive coverage, such as loss owing to breaking glass, theft, fire, or vandalism, and usually subject to a dollar deductible
(2) Collision coverage
(3) Other, such as coverage that insures against towing and labor claims resulting from breakdown of your automobile; usually defined by a dollar limit

8. *Dishonesty insurance*. You should consider insuring yourself against monetary losses suffered at the hands of a dishonest employee. This can be accomplished by the purchase of a fidelity bond. A blanket fidelity bond can be purchased to cover losses suffered at the hands of any worker in your employment without listing the names of specific employees. Fidelity bonds usually cover any dishonest act or criminal act by employees, including theft and embezzlement. The bonds usually cover losses that occur while the bond is in force or for a specified discovery period, usually several years after the bond has been discontinued.

Retirement Plans

You do not have to have an incorporated practice to provide a retirement plan for yourself or your employees. Retirement plans can offer significant tax savings. For an unincorporated, self-employed physician there are several available options. You should obtain the advice of your accountant and attorney about which retirement plan is best suited to your needs and circumstances.

1. *Keogh plan*. The Keogh (pronounced key-oh) plan was named after Congressman Eugene Keogh who introduced the original legislation in Congress in 1962. Since then the original law has been changed several times to keep up with inflation (most recently by the Economic Recovery Tax Act of 1981), but the name Keogh has been retained to designate one form of retirement plan available to self-employed persons and partnerships.

   The law allows a self-employed Keogh plan

participant a maximum contribution and deduction of 15 percent of earned income or $15,000, whichever is least. For example, a self-employed physician with an earned income of $100,000 may contribute $15,000 to a Keogh retirement plan. The contribution represents a tax deduction from net taxable income. The earnings on the invested funds accumulate on a tax-deferred basis until withdrawn. The money may be withdrawn as early as age 59½ but no later than age 70½ without paying a substantial penalty.

A Keogh plan must cover all full-time employees, regardless of age, who have worked one thousand hours a year or more for three or more years. For each employee, you must contribute to the Keogh plan an amount equal to the percent contribution made to your own Keogh account. The maximum amount of earned income taken into account for computing the deduction is $200,000. For example, if your net income is $100,000 and you make the maximum $15,000 contribution to your Keogh plan account (15% of $100,000), you must contribute an amount equal to 15 percent of each eligible employee's annual earned income into his or her Keogh account. Similarly, if your annual earned income is $200,000 and you make the maximum $15,000 contribution to your Keogh account (7.5% of $200,000) you must contribute 7.5 percent of each eligible employee's compensation into his or her Keogh account. An employee who leaves your employment after three years has the right to withdraw his or her funds from the Keogh account.

Investments in a Keogh plan may take a number of forms, including common stocks, preferred stocks, mutual funds, money market funds, treasury notes and bills, United States government agency securities, limited real estate partnerships, passbook savings accounts, and time deposits. The Economic Recovery Tax Act of 1981 prohibits funding a Keogh plan with works of art, antiques, rugs, precious metals, gems, stamps, coins, alcoholic beverages, or other collectibles specified in IRS regulations.

The contribution that you as a physician–employer make into each employee's Keogh plan is a business expense deductible on your income tax return, thereby reducing your net taxable income, as is the contribution that you make for your own retirement account.

2. *Employer-sponsored Individual Retirement Account.* The law allows any business, incorporated or unincorporated, to establish an employer-sponsored Individual Retirement Account (IRA). As a physician-employer you may contribute to your IRA a maximum of $2,000 or 100 percent of your annual earned income, whichever is least. You are not required to contribute anything for your employees. You have total freedom to decide which employees to cover, if any, and which not to cover. If you decide to contribute to an IRA for one of your employees, you have the choice to contribute any amount you wish up to a maximum of $2,000 or 100 percent of the employee's annual earned income, whichever is least.

   Employer-sponsored IRA plans permit additional contributions for a nonworking spouse. A spousal IRA allows you to make additional contributions to provide a retirement plan for both you and your spouse. The maximum contribution is $2,250 per year.

   IRA plans are offered by banks, savings and loan institutions, mutual funds, and other financial institutions. All of the money invested and earned in an IRA accumulates free of income tax until the time of withdrawal. The funds may be withdrawn as a lump sum or in monthly increments as an annuity beginning at age 59½ but not later than age 70½.

3. *Simplified Employee Pension Plan.* With the Revenue Act of 1978, Congress authorized a new type of employer-sponsored IRA known as a *Simplified Employee Pension Plan,* which can be established by any employer, whether incorporated or unincorporated. The contributions allowed to a tax-deferred Simplified Employee Pension Plan are equal to those allowed to a Keogh plan (i.e., 15 percent of your annual

earned income up to a maximum of $15,000). Likewise, the law requires employers to contribute to an employee's Simplified Employee Pension Plan an amount based on the same percentage as the employer contributed to his or her own account. A Simplified Employee Pension Plan, however, differs from a Keogh plan in a number of ways. Some of the major differences are

a. A Simplified Employee Pension Plan must cover all eligible full- and part-time employees.
b. Employees must be at least twenty-five years of age to participate in a Simplified Employee Pension Plan.
c. An employee must have been in your employment for three of the preceding five years to participate in a Simplified Employee Pension Plan.
d. An employee must have earned at least $200 in the year the contribution was made.

Contributions to a Keogh plan, employer-sponsored IRA, or Simplified Employee Pension Plan must be shown on the employee's W–2 form as part of his or her gross income. The contribution represents added income for the employee, but is also wholly deductible on the employee's income tax return as a retirement plan contribution, thus costing the employee nothing in taxes.

4. *Individual Retirement Account.* The Economic Recovery Tax Act of 1981 allows you and your employees, whether enrolled in an IRS-approved, employer-sponsored retirement plan (Keogh, employer-sponsored IRA, Simplified Employee Pension Plan, pension plan, profit sharing plan), to contribute and deduct the lesser of $2,000 or 100 percent of your annual earned income to an IRA. In the case of a spousal IRA, the maximum contribution and deduction is the lesser of $2,250 or 100 percent of annual earned income. As in an employer-sponsored IRA, all of the money invested and earned in your IRA will accumulate income tax free until the time of withdrawal.

The fund may not be withdrawn until age $59^1/_2$ and not later than age $70^1/_2$. The IRS will levy a 10 percent excise penalty on any premature withdrawal unless the reason for withdrawal is death or disability.

Interest Charges and Service Charges

The Judicial Council of the American Medical Association (AMA) has taken the position that it is "not in the best interest of the public or the profession" for a physician to charge interest on an unpaid bill or to charge a penalty or fee for professional fees not paid within a specific period of time. The AMA also indicates that it is not in the best interest of the public or the profession for the physician to charge a collection fee if the account is given to a collection agency. The Judicial Council of the AMA, however, accepts that a physician may add a service charge based on the actual administrative costs of rebilling an account not paid within a reasonable period of time. Patients must be notified in advance of the existence of this practice. You may inform patients of your billing practices by several methods.

1. Include a statement about your service charge in your office information and policy booklet given to patients when they first come to your office
2. Have a statement about service charges printed on each of your end-of-the-month bills
3. Have your patient sign a statement agreeing to pay a service charge on any unpaid balance due beyond a reasonable time limit at the time he or she signs other releases and authorizations when registering as a new patient

Some physicians' offices offer a discount to patients who pay cash for services. If a discount for cash payment is to be offered, it should be intended to reflect the administrative costs of rebilling a patient's account. Discounts and service charges may be subject to federal statutory disclosure under the Federal Truth in Lending Act; state statutes impose further requirements. Before offering a discount, charging interest, or adding a service charge to patient accounts be sure to check with your county medical society's committee on medical ethics as well as your attorney.

Keeping Your Records Organized

Regardless of the method you adopt to keep your records organized, records you keep must be accurate and complete. The following suggestions are given to help you keep your records organized:

1. Organize a filing system. At the beginning of each year, have your office aide prepare and label twelve monthly folders (January through December). As bills arrive in your office, your office aide should place them in a separate folder labeled *Bills to be Paid.* When you pay your bills during the month, your aide should write a check, mark the bill *paid,* and record the date of payment and the check number on the bill. If your office has received an invoice identifying the goods or services, the invoice number should be recorded on the check before the check is sent to the vendor. When your cancelled check returns from the bank, staple the check to the bill and the invoice. Place the stapled documents in the folder for the month in which you received the bank statement, or in the folder for the month in which the check was written, depending on your accountant's preference. You should keep sales slips, invoices, receipts, cancelled checks, and other documents that clearly show income, deductions, and credits.

   Your personal records at home should likewise be organized in file folders and kept separate from your business files. You may adopt a monthly cancelled check file similar to the one used in your office. However, a file system based on tax-deductible categories is probably preferable for use with your personal records. Examples of titles for your personal record file folders might include the following:

   Alimony
   Casualty and theft losses
   Charitable contributions
   Child care contributions
   Credit and charge card interest
   Dentist bills
   Doctor bills

Drug bills	Nursing care bills
Home mortgage interest	Personal loan interest expenses
Hospital expenses	Personal property taxes
Local income taxes	Political contributions
Miscellaneous deductions (safe-deposit box, Keogh trustee fees, educational expenses)	Real estate taxes
Miscellaneous taxes	State income taxes
	Transportation for medical purposes

You may wish to combine your expense categories into five general folders as an alternative method for organizing your personal records: *Medical and Dental Expenses, Taxes, Contributions, Interest,* and *Miscellaneous.*

2. Make a list of all of the members of your management team including your attorney, accountant, banker, stock broker, and insurance representative.
3. Carefully label and put all important documents in a rented safe-deposit box. Items that can be replaced easily need not be stored in your safe-deposit box. These items include insurance policies, cancelled checks, income tax returns, bank books, social security cards, warranties, and burial instructions. Documents that should be stored in a safe-deposit box include

Birth certificates	Stock and bond certificates
Citizenship papers	Important contracts
Marriage certificates	Veteran's papers
Adoption papers	Death certificates
Divorce decrees	Passports
Deeds	Wills
Titles of automobiles	Other special papers

4. Make a master list of all the documents that you have placed in your safe-deposit box.
5. Store your will properly. The original copy is usually kept in your attorney's safe. You should have two additional copies, one of which should be kept in your safe-deposit box and the other at home. Keeping the original copy of the will in your attorney's safe may prevent any legal delays in obtaining this document at the time of death.

6. Prepare an office and home inventory. The best way to make an inventory is to go from room to room in both your office and your home, listing your belongings. You should list how much each item costs, when it was purchased, the model number, brand name, dealer's name, and general description. As you purchase each new item of equipment for your office and as you acquire furnishings for your home, add these items to your inventory list. You should update your inventory every six months. After completing your inventory list, take photographs of the interior of each room in your office and home. If there is a burglary or fire, your inventory list and photographs will help substantiate your losses and your insurance claim.
7. Prepare a record book of the whereabouts of your important papers (Fig. 14). The book should contain a list of your savings and checking accounts, brokerage accounts, the name and branch of the bank where you have your safe-deposit box, the location of your safe-deposit box keys, the combination to your office or home safe, your social security numbers, your insurance policy information, and a list of your credit cards and numbers. Store the record book in a secure location. Consider giving a copy of the record book to your attorney or a trusted family member.
8. Prepare a file, both at home and at the office, for miscellaneous correspondence each year. One correspondence file should be established for incoming correspondence and one for outgoing correspondence. If a large amount of correspondence accumulates on a specific subject, a separate folder should be made specifically for this subject.

Incorporating Your Practice

Most physicians starting in practice establish a sole proprietorship or partnership. State laws, however, allow for the formation of a professional corporation or professional association as a legal business entity. There are advantages and disadvantages to forming a professional corporation.

Husband's name ______________________
Date of birth ______________________
Social Security number ______________________

Wife's name ______________________
Date of birth ______________________
Social Security number ______________________

Child's name ______________________
Date of birth ______________________
Social Security number ______________________

Child's name ______________________
Date of birth ______________________
Social Security number ______________________

BANK ACCOUNTS

Bank name/address	*Account number*

BROKERAGE ACCOUNTS

Brokerage name/address	*Account number*

MUTUAL FUNDS

Fund name/address	*Account number*	*Description*

STOCKS AND BONDS

Company	*Certificate number*	*Description*	*Purchase date*	*Cost*

LIFE INSURANCE POLICIES

Company/ address	*Policy number*	*Face amount*	*Insurance agent*	*Address/ phone*

HEALTH INSURANCE POLICIES

Company/ address	*Policy number*	*Description*	*Insurance agent*	*Address/ phone*

AUTOMOBILE INSURANCE POLICIES

Automobile	*Automobile serial number*	*Company/address*

Policy number	*Policy coverage*	*Insurance agent*	*Address/phone*

Figure 14. Record book.

PROPERTY INSURANCE

Company/ address	Policy number	Description	Insurance agent	Address/ phone

REAL ESTATE

Property location	Description	Owner(s)	Mortgage holder	Address/ phone

Initial purchase price	Depreciation schedule

CEMETERY

Cemetery location	Description of plot (plot number)

RETIREMENT PLAN(S) (KEOGH PLANS AND IRAS)

Where invested	Account number	Address/phone

HARD ASSETS (SILVER, GOLD, GEMS, COLLECTIBLES)

Type	Quality	Quantity	Purchase date	Purchase price

ADVISORS

	Name	Address/phone
Attorney		
Accountant		
Executor		
Trustees		
Physician		
Dentist		
Stockbroker		

CHARGE CARD ACCOUNTS

Charge card	Card number

LOCATION OF IMPORTANT DOCUMENTS

Wills and trusts __________
Cemetery deed __________
Birth certificates __________
Marriage certificates __________
Death certificates __________
Social Security cards __________
Key to safe deposit box __________
Tax records __________

Figure 14. (Continued)

Veteran's papers ______________________
Immunization records ______________________
Automobile title(s) ______________________
Checkbook ______________________
Bank passbooks ______________________
Stock and bond certificates ______________________
Insurance policies ______________________
Funeral and burial instructions ______________________
Combinations to office and home safes ______
OTHER IMPORTANT INFORMATION:
____
____
____

Figure 14. (Continued)

1. The major advantages of incorporation are the following:

    a. As an employee of a professional corporation, you can make a larger contribution to a retirement fund than you can as a self-employed sole proprietor or partner. The doctor who incorporates his or her practice can lower federal income tax liability by making these larger contributions to a corporate retirement fund. You may also shelter these additional assets made to the corporate retirement fund from a possible malpractice judgment (see also Retirement Plans for Corporations, p. 171).
    b. Under certain circumstances, the corporate form of practice may limit personal liability compared to the liability assumed as a sole proprietor or partner. For example, as a corporate stockholder you would not be held responsible for corporate debts or employee negligence. In a partnership, you may be liable jointly with your partner for the debts of the partnership and negligent acts of your employees. The possible advantage of limiting your personal liability by forming a corporation has been debated by attorneys and should be discussed with your own attorney before considering it a potential advantage to incorporation.

c. The corporate form of practice provides the doctor with numerous fringe benefits.

(1) The corporation can pay the medical and dental expenses of its employees and their families. Medical and dental expenses and premiums paid by the corporation for major medical, hospitalization, surgical, and dental insurance plans are deductible from gross income as a corporate expense. Benefits are also tax-free to corporate employees. Employees must fulfill certain requirements to qualify for a medical expense plan. They must be employed as full-time workers, usually defined as working more than twenty hours per week or 1,000 hours per year. Employees must also be at least twenty-five years old and have worked for the corporation for at least three years.

(2) The corporation may pay the premiums for employees' disability insurance. The premiums are deductible by the corporation and provide a tax-free benefit for the employee.

(3) The corporation may pay the premiums for the first $50,000 of group term life insurance as a tax-free benefit for an employee and as an expense deductible from the gross income of the corporation. The corporation may, under certain specific circumstances outlined in the federal tax laws, pay the premiums for higher amounts of insurance (greater than $50,000) on an employee as a corporate expense; however, the employee may be taxed for the portion of the premium above the $50,000 limit.

(4) A professional corporation can own an automobile. It can take an investment credit for the year in which the automobile was purchased, depreciate the automobile, pay for the automobile insurance, repairs, gas, and oil, and rent the car to

you for personal use. Even though you may drive the automobile entirely for professional business matters, the IRS does not permit your corporation to deduct 100 percent of the automobile expenses. The travel between your home and your first business-related stop of the day is not considered deductible. This means that you may not use 100 percent of your automobile expenses for tax deduction purposes. Your accountant should advise you about acceptable methods of determining a percentage deduction for your corporation-owned automobile.

(5) A professional corporation may pay a $5,000 death benefit to the beneficiary of a deceased employee. The death benefit is tax-free to the beneficiary and is a tax-deductible expense to the corporation.

2. Some of the disadvantages of incorporation include the following:

   a. The legal costs for establishing a corporation may be substantial. The costs may include such things as filing fees, stock certificates, minute books, corporate seal, and the drafting of documents such as articles of incorporation, bylaws, employment agreements, retirement plans, and medical-dental reimbursement programs.
   b. The legal expenses for continuing a corporate form of practice may be higher than for a less complex form of business organization. The expenses may arise from such necessities as keeping corporate minutes and drafting additional retirement plan amendments to comply with changing laws.
   c. There are more tax forms to file and paperwork to complete for a corporation, including such things as corporate income tax and retirement plan forms.
   d. Administration of corporate retirement plans will involve additional costs to handle such matters as fidelity bonds and actuarial fees.

Considering that the Economic Recovery Tax Act of 1981 has made it possible for a self-employed physician to contribute $15,000 or 15 percent of annual earned income (whichever is less) to a Keogh plan or Simplified Employer Pension Plan, incorporation may not seem an appealing way to plan for retirement. Unless you anticipate contributing 25 percent of your annual earned income each year toward your retirement, or your income substantially exceeds $100,000, incorporation may not offer attractive advantages. The advantages, disadvantages, and alternatives to incorporation should be discussed with your accountant, attorney, insurance advisor, and professional management consultant to establish which form of practice is best suited to your needs.

Retirement Plans for Corporations

If you are incorporating your practice, or if you are joining an incorporated practice, you should be familiar with the types of retirement plans available for incorporated practices. There are basically two categories of retirement plans used by incorporated practices: *defined contribution* and *defined benefit.*

To understand the difference between a defined contribution plan and a defined benefit plan, consider the following analogy. Imagine you wish to purchase an automobile. You may go to an automobile dealer and explain that your budget will allow you to pay a specific number of defined cash installments to purchase an automobile. With this information, the automobile dealer will tell you what kind of automobile you can purchase with your defined budget. In this example you define your contribution and the dealer tells you the type automobile you can obtain. The defined contribution retirement plan is analogous in that you define the amount of money to contribute to a retirement plan over a set number of years until the date of retirement; the defined contributions plus any earnings on the contributions establish the ultimate benefit.

The alternative to the defined contribution plan

is the defined benefit plan. Consider again the example of purchasing an automobile. This time, you tell the automobile dealer that you wish to purchase a *specific* automobile, and you ask the dealer how much your installment payments must be to obtain it. The automobile dealer will point out that your installment payments will be higher if you wish to purchase the automobile in one year than if you wish to make installment payments over a more prolonged period of time, perhaps three or four years. This example is analogous to a defined benefit retirement plan. The amount of the projected retirement benefit is defined and the annual contribution or installment payments are calculated based on the length of time from initiation of the plan to the date of retirement plus any assumed rate of growth of the invested funds. Although the concept is simple, the calculations for a defined benefit plan require the services of an actuary.

1. *Defined contribution plans.* There are three types of defined contribution plans.

   a. *Profit sharing plan.* A corporation sponsoring a profit sharing retirement plan has no fixed commitment to make or continue annual contributions. Each year the corporate board decides the amount of money to be added to the profit sharing plan based on a percent of the employee's annual earned income. Under current pension laws, the limit on contributions to a profit sharing plan is 15 percent of an employee's annual earned income up to a dollar maximum of $45,475 (in 1982). The law provides for annual adjustments of the maximum dollar contribution to keep pace with inflation.

      An equal percentage of each eligible employee's annual earned income is contributed to a pool of money invested by a trustee. The income earned on the fund accumulates tax free. On reaching retirement age each employee receives his or her share of the fund in either a retirement annuity or a lump sum distribution that is then taxable as ordinary income in the year received.

If the employee leaves the plan by reason of death, disability, or termination of employment, he or she is entitled to a portion (or all) of the contributed funds based on a vesting formula outlined in the trust agreement.

b. *Money purchase plan.* In a money purchase plan, the rate of contribution is fixed at the time the plan is drafted. The percent contribution may not vary from year to year. The corporation must make the contribution in profitable as well as lean years. Under current pension laws, the limitation on contributions to a money purchase plan is 25 percent of an employee's annual earned income up to a dollar maximum of $45,475 (in 1982). The law provides for annual adjustments of the maximum dollar contribution to keep pace with inflation.

c. *Target benefit plan.* A target benefit plan is a hybrid plan with features of both a money purchase plan and a defined benefit plan. A target benefit plan requires an annual corporate contribution. The contribution is calculated on an actuarial basis, like a defined benefit plan. The contribution for an individual, however, cannot exceed 25 percent of the employee's annual earned income up to a dollar maximum of $45,475 (in 1982). A target benefit plan may be used in lieu of a money purchase plan in instances when a physician is much older than other corporate employees and does not wish to establish a defined benefit plan.

A money purchase plan and a profit sharing plan may be combined, allowing for a combined total contribution of 25 percent of an employee's annual earned income up to a dollar maximum of $45,475 (in 1982). Since contributions to a profit sharing plan may be made in any amount up to 15 percent of an employee's annual earned income, a common method for combining the two plans is to provide a fixed 10 percent contribution to a money purchase plan and a flexible contribution up to a maximum of 15 percent of an employee's annual earned income to a profit sharing plan.

2. *Defined benefit plan.* A defined benefit retirement plan defines the amount of the annual retirement benefit available to the participant at the date of retirement. The variables involved in establishing a defined benefit retirement plan include the following:

    a. The amount of annual benefit to be paid at the time of retirement. The law specifies the maximum allowable benefit. Under current pension laws a defined benefit retirement plan can provide an annual retirement benefit to an employee in an amount equal to 100 percent of the employee's annual earned income, but cannot exceed a dollar maximum of $136,425 (in 1982). There is no limit to the annual corporate contribution, only to the benefit payable at the time of retirement. The law provides for annual adjustments of the maximum dollar amount payable at the time of retirement to keep pace with inflation.
    b. The projected annual return on invested funds. The projected annual return on invested funds is usually established by your pension plan advisor in conjunction with an actuary. The projected annual return is usually attainable through conservative investments.
    c. The age of the participant(s) in the retirement plan. The younger the participant, the more retirement plan contributions must be made by the corporation to reach the defined benefit. The more time available for contributions, the smaller dollar amount each contribution needs to be. Likewise, the older the participant(s) and the closer they are to the age of retirement, the larger the retirement plan contributions must be to reach the desired defined benefit by the date of retirement.

Although somewhat more complicated in design and more expensive to establish and administer, it is possible to combine a defined contribution plan and a defined benefit plan to achieve even greater retirement benefits. The pension laws also allow a physician to build up a retirement account even further by making voluntary contributions to a retirement plan out of net income in an amount equal to 6 percent of his or her annual earned income. Under certain specific circumstances outlined in the retirement laws, this voluntary contribution may be as much as ten percent.

The present pension laws provide incorporated practices with a wide variety of retirement options to choose from. The retirement option(s) that you select will depend on your age, the age of other corporate employees, the age of other physicians in the corporate retirement plan, the amount of money you wish to accumulate for your retirement, and the degree of flexibility you wish to have in making contributions to your retirement plan. You should consult your tax advisor about the best retirement plan(s) to meet your specific needs.

Handling Your Funds

When you begin your practice, you should open two checking accounts: a checking account for business expenditures and a checking account for personal expenditures. At the same time, you should open a savings account for your practice. The savings account may be at the same bank as your checking account or at another bank or savings institution. Savings and loan institutions and savings banks are allowed by law to pay a higher interest rate than savings accounts in a commercial bank. Wherever you open your savings account, make sure that you will earn daily interest from date of deposit to date of withdrawal.

You should keep the minimum amount in your office checking account that avoids a service charge. All your practice receipts should be deposited into your savings account to earn daily interest. When your office aide writes checks, usually twice a month, the amount of money required to pay the checks can be transferred to your checking account. Many financial institutions allow you to transfer funds by telephone from one account to another or from one financial institution to another. When you open your savings account for your practice, consider opening another savings account for your personal funds.

1. *Personal funds*

   a. *Bank accounts.*

      (1) *Bank savings account.* A savings account may be opened at the same bank in which you have your personal checking account. Money deposited in a savings account can be withdrawn at any time and is insured for up to $100,000 by the federal government.

      (2) *NOW account.* A NOW account can be opened at a commercial bank, a savings and loan institution, or a savings bank. A NOW account combines an interest-bearing account with check-writing features. Most NOW accounts have minimum balance requirements. The minimum varies from institution to institution. The NOW account allows deposits and check writing on one account. If you establish a NOW account, you should avoid leaving excess cash in the account. The extra accumulated cash should be reinvested in higher-yielding, liquid assets such as treasury bills, short-term certificates of deposit, or money market funds. Many financial institutions that offer NOW accounts differ widely in their minimum cash requirements, service charges, and convenience. Commercial banks usually have higher minimum cash requirements to open a NOW account but may have more branches located conveniently near your office, longer banking hours, and drive-in windows.

          There may be substantial service charges and penalties if your NOW account does not meet the minimum balance requirements. Some institutions make a service charge for balances that fall below a minimum on a single day in any month, whereas others judge the minimum on the basis of your average daily balance throughout the month. Some banks and savings institutions make special per-check charges in addition to service charges as a penalty for failing to meet the monthly minimum balance; others penalize you a part or all of the interest earned in your account for the month.

If a NOW account requires a high minimum cash reserve and has significant service charges and penalties, you may find it more convenient and profitable to maintain a regular checking account and keep the cash that would have been required to fund the minimum balance for a NOW account invested in higher-yielding, liquid assets as noted earlier.

Most lending institutions offer NOW accounts for personal checking accounts but not for corporate or business accounts.

(3) *Savings and loan savings account.* The interest rate allowed by federal law in a savings account at a savings and loan or savings bank institution is one-quarter percent more than can be paid by a commercial bank on a savings account. As with a commercial bank savings account, the money is federally insured up to $100,000 and can be withdrawn at any time without penalty.

b. *Cash management services.* A cash management service represents an all-in-one combination of a checking account, money market investment, stock and bond portfolio, and credit card account. Merrill Lynch pioneered this financial service and offers the prototype, Cash Management Account. Subscribers to the Merrill Lynch Cash Management Account pay an annual fee ($28 in 1982), and must deposit $20,000 in cash, securities, or both to open the account. Accounts are insured up to $500,000. Interest and dividends paid on securities, proceeds from the sale of securities, and additional deposits are all automatically invested in a money market fund.

Subscribers may withdraw their funds from the money market fund by writing a check. Checks may be written against the account balance in any amount. This is an advantage over most money market funds, which limit check withdrawals to a minimum of $500 or $1,000. The Cash Management Account offers a VISA credit card free of charge. Charges on the VISA card are paid directly from funds in the holder's money market account. Subscribers who do not have a credit balance in their money market accounts may borrow against their securities.

Cash Management Account subscribers receive a monthly detailed statement of all account activity and the price of their securities. For an additional annual fee, Merrill Lynch subscribers have the right to shift into a tax-exempt money market fund.

A number of other brokerage firms offer similar cash management services and are listed in Appendix 31.

c. *Money market funds*. Money market funds are portfolios of high-interest-bearing securities sold to investors as a mutual fund. The securities are usually treasury bills, federal paper, commercial paper, and certificates of deposit on United States banks and branches of United States banks in foreign countries. Checks can usually be written against these accounts. The amount of the check usually must exceed a certain minimum amount.

The funds vary in terms of portfolio maturity, types of investments, and even by quality of investments. Investments made in money market funds are not federally insured. Although the larger funds are generally sound, it is advisable for you to review the fund's portfolio of investments before investing.

Donoghue's Money Market Fund Directory is a complete and comprehensive text about money market funds with a listing of all the funds. This book may be obtained by writing to *Donoghue's Money Market Fund Directory*, Post Office Box 540, Holliston, Massachusetts 01746. Some of the larger institutions that offer money market funds are listed in Appendix 32.

2. *Handling cash surplus from your practice.* As your practice deposits exceed your monthly practice expenses (including the payment of salaries), and as a cash surplus accumulates in your practice savings account, you should consider transferring the surplus funds from your relatively low-interst-bearing savings account into a higher-interest-bearing investment. The interest rates on the following investments are published daily in the *Wall Street Journal,* 200 Burnett Road, Chicopee, Massachusetts 01021, and in other financial news sources.

    a. *Savings certificates.* Savings certificates are time deposits offered by savings institutions and usually pay more interest than a passbook savings account. Savings certificates are insured by the federal government. Maturities vary from thirty days to many years. If you purchase a savings certificate, the certificate should have a short maturity in terms of months so you can have the funds available if you should need them quickly (liquidity). If the money is withdrawn before the savings certificate matures, there is a penalty involving a substantial loss of interest.
    b. *United States treasury bills.* United States treasury bills (T-Bills) are securities sold by the federal government to finance the national debt. They offer the maximum degree of liquidity and safety of any investment since they are backed by the full faith and credit of the United States treasury. United States treasury bills are issued in minimum denominations of $10,000 and in additional $5,000 increments. The interest on a treasury bill is not taxed by state or local governments. Treasury bills have a maturity ranging from three months to one year. The treasury bills

maturing in three months and six months are offered at auction every Monday. Twelve-month treasury bills are offered once every four weeks. The interest rate paid on treasury bills changes depending on the results of the auction. Treasury bills may be purchased for a small fee (usually $25 to $40) from a commercial bank or other financial institutions including some brokerage firms; or they may be purchased directly from the United States Treasury without a service fee by submitting an order (noncompetitive bid) to the Federal Reserve Bank in your district (see Appendix 30). Further information about United States treasury bills may be obtained from the Bureau of the Public Debt, Securities Transaction Branch, Washington, D.C. 20226.

c. *Money market certificates.* These certificates are six-month, government-insured time deposits offered by banks and savings institutions. The interest rate offered on a money market certificate varies from week to week and is established at one-quarter percent above the interest rate for treasury bills. The minimum investment is $10,000 and there is a penalty for early withdrawal.
d. *Money market funds.* (See discussion of money market funds listed under savings accounts for your personal money, section 1.c.)
e. *Commercial paper.* Commercial paper represents short-term corporate borrowings that are not backed by any collateral. The safety of commercial paper depends on the financial soundness of the corporation issuing the corporate paper. Maturities vary from thirty days to a year or more. The minimum investment is usually $100,000.

Float

Financial institutions and industry have long recognized that it is profitable to let other people's money work for them. One variation of this principle is known as *float.* You do not have to be a large financial institution to use the same principle in your own personal and professional management. Here is how to use float and earn additional interest at no additional cost.

1. Pay your debt obligations on time. You do not, however, have to pay your bills before they are due. Send a check a day or two before they are due. By paying this way, you keep your money earning maximum interest for you for as long as possible.
2. Consider paying your debt obligations with a check drawn on a money market fund or bank geographically remote from your community. Your money will continue earning interest for several additional days while your check goes through the Federal Reserve System and is finally deducted from your money market fund or bank account. If you pay your bills consistently in this way, the additional interest you will earn will add up over the year. You should consider paying your mortgage installments, local, state, and federal taxes, insurance premiums, and all other major items of indebtedness in this fashion.
3. Charge all possible expenditures, personal and professional, to a credit card. Your credit card charges should be paid on time but not more than a few days before they are due.
4. Have your accountant calculate the minimum that you need to withdraw in withholding tax from your salary paychecks. Make sure the amount withdrawn complies with IRS regulations without incurring a penalty. Generally, you are not required to withhold more than 80 percent of your estimated tax liability based on your previous year's salary. On April 15 you will owe the government the remaining tax liability. Invest the money that would have been paid to the government as withholding tax in a short-term treasury bill, a certificate of deposit, or a money market fund. Collect the interest, and on April 14 send in your check for the balance of your tax liability.

Contributions to Charity

As a respected and responsible member of your community, you will be expected to make donations to numerous charitable causes. It is difficult for you to know the financial and ethical reliability of a charitable organization. There are some charities that advertise themselves as worthy causes, whereas most of the donation goes to pay the salaries of the fund raisers and the advertising costs.

1. *Choosing a charity*. If you have a question about a charitable organization you may obtain in-depth information about the charity (excluding fraternal, religious, and political organizations) from the National Information Bureau, 419 Park Avenue South, New York, New York 10016. Your Better Business Bureau can also provide information about local charities as well as a list of any complaints that have been made about charitable organizations in your area. If you do not have a Better Business Bureau, you may write to the Council of Better Business Bureaus, 1150 Seventeenth Street, NW, Washington, D.C. 20036, for specific information about a charity.

   The Philanthropic Advisory Service, a division of the Council of Better Business Bureaus, monitors and reports on national and international soliciting organizations. The Philanthropic Advisory Service publishes a newsletter (*Insight*) featuring news briefs and articles of general interest in the philanthropic field. Subscriptions may be obtained by writing to the Philanthropic Advisory Service, Council of Better Business Bureaus, 1515 Wilson Boulevard, Arlington, Virginia 22209 (703-276-0100).

   The Philanthropic Advisory Service also publishes a quarterly update on charitable, educational, and religious organizations and lists those organizations whose practices meet the voluntary standards recommended by the Better Business Bureau. This update includes the public disclosure of such things as

   a. Activities and finances
   b. Compensation of the governing board of the charitable organization and details about its decision-making structure
   c. Financial accountability including the percentage of total income spent directly on pro-

gram services as distinct from fund-raising and administrative costs

d. Fund-raising practices

e. Accuracy and truthfulness of solicitations and informational materials

The Philanthropic Advisory Service also lists those organizations from which the Council of Better Business Bureaus has requested information regarding governance, fund raising, and financial information on three separate occasions, and that have failed to comply with voluntary disclosure.

2. *Some guidelines for giving to charity.* You should consider the following charity-giving suggestions:

   a. The IRS requires proof of payment if you claim a charitable donation for tax purposes. Always try to get a receipt for your donation. To guarantee proof that you made the contribution, write a check for your donation. Your cancelled check may be your only form of receipt.
   b. Avoid giving to unknown charities solicited by someone on a street corner with a canister and a brochure.
   c. Avoid putting cash in charity boxes near the cash registers of local merchants. In some instances these donations never reach the charitable organization.
   d. Prepare an annual budget for your charitable donations, which may include such things as

      (1) Church
      (2) United Way
      (3) Fraternal organizations
      (4) Political candidates and organizations
      (5) Educational institutions
      (6) Other

   e. Never commit yourself to a charitable contribution to an unknown caller on the telephone. If an individual solicits a charitable contribution from you on the telephone, ask that the information about the charity be sent to you in the mail for you to review first. If there is any question about the financial or ethical reliability of the organization, write to the National Information Bureau or the Council of Better Business Bureaus. Try to send your check for a charitable contribution directly to the national office of the charity.

f. Whether your practice is incorporated or unincorporated, write all checks for charitable contributions out of your personal checking account rather than your business checking account to obtain a tax deduction on your personal income taxes.

g. If you make a contribution other than cash to a charitable organization and plan to deduct the contribution from your income tax return, be sure to obtain a reliable appraisal of the current fair market value of your contribution and consider attaching the appraisal to your income tax return.

7. Billing and Collections

Professional Fees

There is no set fee for every medical service, for every medical community, or for every medical situation. The key to establishing your professional fees is to charge the "going rate" for your community. The following may help you establish the "going rate" in your practice situation:

1. The California Medical Association Relative Value Study is a valuable source. This study assigns a relative value scale to all medical and surgical services. For example, an appendectomy may have a relative value scale of 3, a cholecystectomy a relative value scale of 8, a sigmoidoscopy a relative value scale of 0.3, and an internist's complete physical examination a relative value scale of 0.65. It is then up to the physician to designate an actual monetary value for each relative value unit, and calculate fees for each particular service on this basis. A relative value scale gives you some established rational basis on which to set your fees.

   You are not bound by the relative value scale. Obviously, you can make any alterations to fit your practice and skills, but this system does provide a set of general guidelines. Relative value studies have been duplicated in other states using the California Relative Value Study format.
2. Consult health insurers and health agency fee schedules. Examples of these schedules include the Metropolitan Life Insurance Company schedule, Prudential Life Insurance Company schedule, and the department of health and rehabilitative services fee schedule. One schedule that deserves special attention is the third-party insurance carrier, Blue Shield. You should contact the Blue Shield service office in your area and inquire about guidelines for professional fees.

   Each Medicare intermediary maintains a fee profile of physician charges for all services performed by every doctor in its locality who bills a Medicare recipient. Medicare intermediaries screen all charges for all procedures and determine the seventy-fifth percentile of charges as the prevailing charge for a procedure. Medicare intermediaries pay 80 percent of the prevailing charge or 80 percent of the doctor's usual charge (customary charge), whichever is less. The prevailing charge is recomputed and updated on July 1 each year (see also Insurance Claims, p. 109).

A physician going into practice does not have an established fee profile. The Medicare intermediary reimburses physicians newly in practice on the basis of the fiftieth percentile of the usual charges (prevailing charges) of physicians in the same specialty and location. A physician must accumulate three months of charge data in any calendar year to establish his or her own usual or customary charge for a procedure. A physician who begins practice after October 1 in any year will therefore be reimbursed at the fiftieth percentile until July 1 of the second calendar year that follows (i.e., twenty-one months later).

Under the Federal Truth and Information Act you are allowed to obtain a copy of your fee profile and compare it to the prevailing charges in your locality. You should write to your Medicare intermediary on July 1 each year for this information.

Publish your fee schedule once you have established it. Publication means typing the schedule and making it available for all your office aides to refer to easily and show to your patients if they request it. Several years ago when President Nixon imposed wage and price controls, it was mandatory to conspicuously display a physician's fee schedule or post a notice stating that all professional fees were available for inspection. It is not mandatory now to openly display your fee schedule; however, it is still a good idea to have such a list readily available for review. Patients may call and inquire about professional fees. Having a printed list of fees available helps your aides answer such inquiries. A printed list of fees also counters the often-heard complaint that doctors charge whatever they think the patient can afford.

Billing Patients for Outside Laboratory Tests

As a convenience for your patients, you may wish to draw blood specimens in your office, process them, and send them to a local laboratory or mail them to an out-of-town laboratory for processing. To avoid ethical problems, consider billing the patient for a professional service fee related to the drawing and processing of the blood sample rather than establishing a commission, profit, or mark-up on the laboratory fees. If you are not performing the laboratory work in your office and are billing the patient for a drawing and processing charge, the patient should be notified that a separate bill will be sent by the laboratory.

Collecting Your Professional Fees

The keys to successful collection of professional fees are to educate your patients to make payments at the time services are rendered, to project your expectations that these payments will be made by providing visual clues and handing patients their bills, and finally to have a firm, aggressive collection policy implemented by your front office personnel.

1. *Point of service payment.* The ideal solution to collecting patient accounts is to receive point of service payment, a method that eliminates all future collection problems. Although not all patients will be able to pay their bills at the time service is delivered, you can design a system that encourages them to do so. The following guidelines are recommended to promote point of service payment:

    a. Educate your patients about fee policies when first office visits are scheduled. Many doctors' offices inform patients arranging their first appointments that professional fees are to be paid by cash, check, or credit card at the completion of each office visit.

    b. Give your patients written notice of your office policy. Your office policy booklet should include a section that discusses your office fee policy. You should state that point of service payment will be expected unless special arrangements are made in advance with your office personnel.

c. Give your patients visual clue reinforcements regarding your office collection policy. A small, discrete sign may be placed in a conspicuous area of your reception room reminding patients that it is customary and expected that professional services will be paid for when rendered, and that any other method of payment must be arranged in advance. Place a small placard at the checkout window where your patients present bills for payment. The placard should read, "Make checks payable to (doctor's name) ."

d. Project your expectations that patients will make point of service payment. After delivery of services, the doctor should complete the patient's billing form indicating the services rendered and circling the fees. The doctor should hand the itemized bill directly to the patient and ask the patient to take the bill to the front office on leaving.

e. Have your office personnel project their expectations of point of service payment. When patients return itemized bills to your front office personnel, they should be told the dollar amount of the professional fees for that day's service and be asked if they will be paying by cash or by check. No other alternative should be given at that time.

If patients cannot make total payment, partial payment should be sought. If they cannot make any payment at the time service is rendered, your office aide should obtain a firm commitment regarding the exact time when payment might be expected. The promised date of payment should be recorded in an obvious fashion, and your aide should verbally reconfirm the date. Patients should be given a stamped envelope with your office address on it in which to return payment. If patients do not return payment on the promised date, your office aide should call and indicate that payment has not been received.

2. *End-of-the-month billing.* Most physicians bill unpaid accounts at the end of each month. The following guidelines are given to aid you in collecting payment by end-of-the-month billing:

   a. Mail your end-of-the-month bills so that they reach the patient one or two days before the first day of the month. Bills that are received first by the patient have a greater chance of being paid at the beginning of the month before the patient's allocated bill-paying budget is exhausted.
   b. Consider using colored stationery and envelopes for end-of-the-month bills. Studies indicate that a colored envelope catches the attention of the recipient better than a white envelope and therefore has a greater chance of being paid first.
   c. Establish a fast, effective collection procedure. Speed and regularity are the keys to any successful billing collection procedure. The average overdue account depreciates rapidly unless regular communication is established between the doctor-creditor and the patient-debtor. Time becomes a refuge for the debtor looking for a reason to delay or ignore his or her credit obligation.
   d. Send the bill to the patient in a return, self-addressed envelope. These so-called round trip envelopes, which incorporate the bill and a self-addressed envelope, may be purchased from local printing companies or business office suppliers. There are a number of commercial medical printing companies and companies that specialize in business systems that also sell round-trip envelopes (see Appendix 24).
   e. Keep the patient aware of the progress of your collection of insurance benefits. Send the patient a monthly statement and indicate on the billing statement by stamp or adhesive sticker that insurance processing is still in progress and that a final bill will be sent to the patient for any balance due after insurance benefits have been received. Once your office has received the patient's insurance

benefits, your office personnel should initiate your routine billing collection program to collect any remaining balance due on the patient's account. If your office does not file for a patient's insurance benefits (i.e., does not accept assignment), the routine billing collection system should be initiated immediately.

Table 3 suggests a system for routine billing of patient accounts, excluding those patients who are involved in legal proceedings, have special insurance problems, or are in financial difficulties and have made arrangements with your office.

3. *Preparing end-of-the-month bills.* There are several ways to prepare your end-of-the-month bills.

   a. If you have a small number of end-of-the-month statements (less than 50), your office aide can prepare an individually typed, itemized statement of the patient's account.
   b. If you have an office copy machine, a copy of the patient's account receivable card may be duplicated and sent as an end-of-the-month statement. Most physicians who use the pegboard accounting system will use some variant of this method to bill unpaid accounts.
   c. You may use billing services that operate copy vans. The copy van operator duplicates your accounts receivable cards and does the additional work of stuffing, sealing, and stamping your statements on the premises.
   d. You may use a variation of the copy van service, the microfilm service. A representative of a billing service brings a portable microfilm camera to your office and photographs your accounts receivable cards. The film is mailed to the billing company laboratory where it is developed. Statements are then prepared and mailed. One of the companies that offers this service is Creative Systems, Post Office Box 338–209 Franklin, Cedar Falls, Iowa 50613 (319-266-3531). In 1982 the average cost of using a microfilm billing service was about twenty-five cents per statement, plus postage. The charge may vary based on

factors such as the time of the month that the bill is mailed, the volume of statements mailed, the use of special color envelopes, the insertion of collection letters or educational material, the preparation of a logo for your billing envelopes, and the use of postage stamps rather than metering.

e. You may use a computer service company to provide monthly billing. Many of these companies can also program their computers to analyze your accounts receivable; calculate your income statement; prepare payroll forms; report a daily log of charges and payments; report monthly production of total charges, payments, and credits; prepare insurance forms and ledger cards; analyze accounts receivable with report of accounts over 90 days old; generate collection letters; and provide recall notices.

There are two basic methods to provide the computer service center with your office data. The first method is *batch processing* and consists of mailing or delivering to the computer center all the collected financial data on a daily basis. The patient's accounts receivable records are updated at one time. The disadvantage to this method is that your office cannot provide a patient with his or her current balance except at those intervals when the computer updates the patient's account receivable card. Computer service bureaus that use batch processing bill on the basis of production at a flat rate such as fifty cents per statement. There may be additional charges for initial computer programming, supplies, typesetting, and stationery.

The second method used to provide the computer service center with your office data is by means of an office terminal connected to the computer. Your information is transmitted over your office terminal to the computer by a telephone connection. The computer can recall data required and transmit it back to your office, reproducing the data on a teletypewriter. Computer service bureaus

Table 3. Suggested Billing Collection System

Month	Date	Action taken
Date of service rendered	January 15	Send itemized statement
End of the month in which service was rendered	January 29	Send routine end-of-the-month statement to reach the patient by the first of the month
2	February 28	Send end-of-the-month statement with a simple message stamped or applied by adhesive sticker that the account is 30 days overdue[1]
3	March 29	Send end-of-the-month statement with a more forceful message that the account remains overdue, requesting the patient to make immediate payment[2]
4	April 15	Have your office personnel make attempts to contact the patient by telephone to discuss immediate payment of the overdue bill
4	April 28	Send an end-of-the-month statement with a final notice stamped or applied by adhesive sticker indicating that if the account is not paid within 15 days further collection steps will be taken[3]
5	May 15	Send a certified letter to the patient indicating that care is terminated and advising that one of the following actions may be taken:[4] The account may be turned over to a collection agency A suit may be filed in the small claims court The account may be turned over to a debt collection attorney (the signed postal acknowledgement that the patient has received the certified letter should be received in your office to verify the patient's address and validate that the patient has been legally put on notice before further action is taken)
5	May 31	The following alternatives are available: Turn the account over to a collection agency File a claim in the small claims court Turn the account over to a debt collection attorney Write off the account as a bad debt

[1] Example: "Our office records show that your account is overdue. Your prompt payment will be greatly appreciated." Note: Most local business supply companies can provide custom-made stamps, and custom-designed stickers can be ordered from your printer. A variety of mass-produced ad-

that use a terminal system usually charge a monthly rental fee for the office terminal. There may be additional charges for computer time, programming fees, rental of interface equipment, and telephone line charges.

A directory of computer consulting services may be obtained from the Independent Computer Consultant Association, Post Office Box 27412, St. Louis, Missouri 63141 (314-567-9708). Computer service bureaus may be found in the yellow pages of the telephone book.

Before you establish your debt collection policies, you should familiarize yourself with the laws of your state concerning collections and harassment of debtors. A helpful reference dealing with this topic entitled *Harassment and Other Collection Taboos* may be obtained from the National Association of Credit Managers, 475 Park Avenue, New York, New York 10016 (see also Collecting Delinquent Accounts).

Collecting Delinquent Accounts

When a patient is delinquent in the payment of his or her account and your business office has exhausted the usual steps for collection (reminder notices, telephone calls), you have several remaining options.

---

hesive stickers with collection messages for delinquent accounts can be purchased from various medical stationery companies (see Appendix 24).

[2] Example: "Our office records show that your account remains overdue. Your account has been due since ________. If there are considerations we should know about please write or call us. Otherwise we shall anticipate your immediate payment by return mail."

[3] Example: "Your account has now been delinquent since ________. Please consider this your final notice. Unless we receive payment or arrangements for payment are made within 15 days, this account will be turned over for collection."

[4] The Federal Fair Debt Collection Practices Act (United States Code title 15, section 1692e) provides that a creditor may advise a consumer (patient) of the possibility of legal action as long as the action is taken or is likely to be taken if the debtor (patient) does not pay the debt. The creditor (doctor) may not, however, threaten either directly or indirectly to take legal action that is not going to be taken or not likely to be taken without risking being sued by the debtor (patient).

1. You may wish to employ a collection agency. There are many agencies that specialize in the collection of medical and dental accounts. In some areas the local medical society may operate a collection service. It is important that you select an ethical collection agency with a good reputation. The following guidelines will help you select a good agency:

   a. Obtain a list of recommended agencies from

      Medical/Dental/Hospital Bureaus of America
      111 E. Wacker Dr.
      Chicago, IL 60601

      Associated Credit Bureaus of America
      Collection Division
      6767 Southwest Freeway
      Houston, TX 77074

      American Collectors Association
      4040 W. Seventieth St.
      Minneapolis, MN 55435

   b. Check with your local medical society for the name of a reliable collection agency.
   c. Check with the Better Business Bureau for any complaints registered against a collection agency that you might consider using.
   d. Check the promptness with which the agency settles for money collected.
   e. Review the collection methods and the type of collection reminders, notices, and letters that a collection agency uses. Make sure that these methods comply with the Federal Fair Debt Collection Practices Act (United States Code title 15, sections 1692–1693). Some of the highlights of that legislation include the following:

      (1) Debt collectors are prohibited from communicating with a patient-debtor at unusual times or places. For example, a debt collector may not make contact with the debtor before 8 A.M. or after 9 P.M.
      (2) If a patient-debtor is represented by an attorney, the debt collector must deal with the attorney.
      (3) A debt collector may not communicate

with a patient-debtor at the patient-debtor's place of employment if the debt collector knows that the patient-debtor's employer prohibits such contact.

(4) If the patient-debtor notifies the debt collector in writing that he or she refuses to pay a bill or no longer wishes any further communication, the debt collector must stop any further communications with the patient-debtor except to explain the possible consequences to the debtor.

(5) Harassment and abusive techniques are prohibited, including the use of threat, violence, or criminal means to harm the patient-debtor's person, reputation, or property; the use of obscene language; the publication of a list of patient-debtors who refuse to pay their debts; and the use of repeated or harassing telephone calls made with the intent to annoy the patient-debtor.

(6) Use of false or misleading representation is prohibited, such as false representations that the debt collector is an attorney; threats to take any action that cannot legally be taken or that is not intended to be taken; threats to communicate false credit information; and use of any written communication that simulates or is falsely represented to be a document authorized or approved by a federal or state court or official agency, intending to create a false impression as to its source, authorization, or approval.

(7) Unfair practices are prohibited, including collecting an additional fee not authorized by law or the terms of the debt agreement; charging the patient-debtor with collect calls or telegram fees; and accepting a check postdated by more than five days except under specified written conditions.

f. Find out the track record of the collection agency (i.e., what percentage of the accounts the agency collects).

g. Find out the collection fee charged by the collection agency. The collection fee may range from 20 to 50 percent of the bill, and may vary according to individual agreements.
h. Do not sign a contract. Most collection agencies do not require a signed contract. If your selected agency insists on a contract, have your attorney review the contract with you before you sign it.

2. You may decide to turn your delinquent patient accounts over to a law firm that specializes in debt collection. There are several published lists containing the names of attorneys who regularly handle claims of creditors, including the following:

   American Directory of Collection Agencies and Attorneys
   The Service Publishing Company
   Washington Building
   Fifteenth and New York Avenues, NW
   Washington, DC 20005

   Clearing House Quarterly
   The Attorney Clearing House Co.
   P.O. Box 8688
   Naples, FL 33941

   Credit Union Attorney Legal Directory
   Legal Directory, Inc.
   110 S. McDonough St.
   Montgomery, AL 36103

   Handling of your patients' delinquent accounts by a law firm specializing in debt collection has the advantage that the law firm can usually go further with legal prosecution than a collection agency. Although many of your patients' delinquent accounts can be handled by your office personnel in the small claims court, an attorney will be required in cases that involve large sums of money or complicated legal procedures, such as garnishment or claims against a bankrupt patient.

   The debt collection attorney may seek to satisfy a creditor's claim by obtaining a writ of garnishment. A writ of garnishment allows the physician-creditor to collect money that may be owed to the patient by a third person (e.g., wages owed by an employer or sums owed in exchange for goods or services). The laws relating to garnishment vary from state to state. In some states, such as Florida, Texas, and California, the law is complicated, and a writ of garnishment for an employee's wages may be difficult to obtain. Garnishment of a federal employee's wages for the satisfaction of professional fees is presently not allowed in any state.

Subchapter II of the Federal Consumer Credit Protection Act (United States Code title 15, sections 1671–1677) places limitations on the amount of a debtor's wages that can be subject to garnishment. The federal law provides that the maximum amount of wages or salaries that may be subject to a writ of garnishment is the lesser of

a. Twenty-five percent of the debtor's disposable net earnings per week remaining after withholding deductions required by law
b. The difference between the debtor's disposable (net) weekly earnings and thirty times the federal minimum hourly wage in effect at the time the wages are payable

For example, if an employee has net weekly earnings of $160, 25 percent of these earnings would be $40. In 1982 the federal minimum wage was $3.35, and thirty times the federal minimum wage is $100.50. The difference between the net weekly earnings ($160) and thirty times the minimum wage ($100.50) would be $59.50. In this example, only $40 of the debtor's wages, the lesser of the two calculated figures, would be subject to a writ of garnishment.

Attorneys that specialize in debt collection are knowledgeable about state and federal laws dealing with garnishments and can advise you about this method of debt collection.

3. You may wish to take your claim for a delinquent bill to a small claims court. These courts have been established to handle claims involving small sums of money. One advantage to the use of a small claims court is that you can use the court without having to hire an attorney. A second advantage is that it is unnecessary for

you, the physician, to appear in the small claims court. Your office aide may appear on your behalf. Your office aide should bring to the hearing the complete medical and office financial records of the patient. Generally, your office records will be accepted by the court at face value.

A simple claim form is usually filed with the small claims court along with a copy of the delinquent bills. You will probably have to pay a small filing fee when you file your claim. The filing fees vary from state to state and from county to county within a state. The filing fee may also vary according to the amount of the claim (see Appendix 25).

The court will usually send a copy of the claim form by certified mail, summoning the debtor to appear for a hearing. The court will notify you if the summons returns unclaimed. You may elect to have it served by the sheriff or another court-appointed officer. The court may charge you an additional fee for hand delivery of the summons. If you practice as a sole proprietor, the claim will be filed in your name as owner of the practice. If you file on behalf of an incorporated practice, the corporation is listed as the plaintiff, and the claim is signed by the corporate officer or by the person authorized by your corporate bylaws to file claims for the corporation. Some states (e.g., Arizona, Illinois, and Wisconsin) require that a corporation be represented by an attorney. Once the debtor has received a summons to appear in the small claims court, he or she has a number of options.

a. The claim may be paid in full. Payment should include the amount of your delinquent bill plus any court costs or additional fees paid for the service of a summons.
b. A document may be signed by the patient stipulating that partial payments will be made until the debt is paid in full. If a debtor signs a stipulation and fails to comply with the terms of the stipulation, your right to return to small claims court without refiling a claim is usually preserved.

Whenever physician and patient agree that the payment of the bill will be made in more than four installments, whether the patient is negotiating installment payments on the bill for an office visit or signing a stipulation to pay a delinquent bill, the Federal Truth in Lending Regulations (United States Code title 15, sections 226.1–226.1503) apply. Regulation Z of the law requires written disclosure of all information including the finance charges. The disclosure document must show

(1) Total amount of the payment due (fee for service)
(2) Down payment, if any
(3) Unpaid balance
(4) Amount financed
(5) Finance or service charges (with the word *finance* or *service* in larger letters than the rest of the surrounding print, as specified by law)
(6) Finance charge expressed as the annual percent of interest
(7) Total dollar amount of the payments (item 4 plus item 5)
(8) Deferred payments (item 1 plus item 5)
(9) Date of each payment
(10) Amount of each payment
(11) Date of the final payment

Several of the medical printing stationery companies have prepared forms for installment payments that comply with the requirements of the Federal Truth in Lending Regulations. Examples of such companies include Colwell, Histacount, and Medical Arts Press (see Appendix 24).

c. The claim may be ignored. In this case you will receive a judgment against the debtor by default. Receiving a judgment gives you the legal right to attach a debtor's assets, including bank accounts, personal accounts, life insurance, stocks, bonds, jewelry, and real property. The state laws define which assets may be attached. Generally, the court will not act as a collection agency on your behalf. It may be necessary for you to hire an attorney to establish the extent of the debtor's assets and execute judgment.

The small claims court will provide you with information on executing your judgment. In many states you may file your judgment in the records of the courthouse. This record serves as a permanent blemish on the debtor's credit record and usually serves as a cloud or defect on the title to any real property the debtor may sell in the county where the judgment is filed. If the debtor satisfies the judgment, you may be required to complete a *satisfaction of judgment* form for the debtor to file with the small claims court, which then clears his or her credit record and the lien against his or her real property.

d. The debtor may appear for the hearing and dispute the claim or file a counterclaim, in which case the court may require that a formal complaint be filed in a higher court. In this case both parties will usually be required to obtain representation by attorneys.

State laws about small claims courts vary widely, defining various dollar limits within the jurisdiction of the court, the number of times the court may be used within a year's time, and the various rights of the parties obtaining judgments. Your attorney should advise you on your specific state statutes.

Tracing the Skipped Patient

A patient with a delinquent bill who leaves town or cannot be found is commonly known as a *skip*. One can usually suspect a skip when your office receives an unopened envelope returned undelivered by the post office. There are a number of things that can be done to help trace a skipped patient:

1. All of your end-of-the-month statement envelopes and letterhead envelopes should be preprinted with the words *Address Correction Re-*

quested appearing below your return address in the upper left-hand corner of the envelope. The post office will search their records and forward the mail, if possible. If a new address is known to the post office, this information will be given to you. There is a small charge made for this service when you receive the information about the corrected address in your office.

2. Have your office aide call the patient's nearest relative and inquire about the patient's new address. The patient's nearest relative should be listed on the initial registration or history form that the patient completed at the time of his or her first office visit. If the skipped patient was seen in consultation in the hospital, the same type of information should be available on the patient's hospital admission records.
3. Call the patient's employer and request the patient's address and telephone number. Make sure that your office aide does not indicate to the employer that the request is in reference to a bad debt. Discussing a patient's delinquent account with his or her employer may be in violation of both state and federal laws related to harassment of debtors.
4. Check the patient's driver's license number on his or her initial registration or history form. Write or call the state motor vehicle bureau and inquire whether the patient has an up-to-date driver's license. You must include the patient's full name and date of birth. If the motor vehicle bureau has a driver's license registration, it will usually send a copy of it to you. This response may provide your office with a new address for the missing debtor.
5. Find out if the patient owns a vehicle registered in your state. You must include the patient's full name and date of birth with your inquiry. The registry of motor vehicles will usually send a copy of a patient's vehicle registration to your office, which may show the patient's current address.
6. Large metropolitan areas have city directories that list street addresses and the persons that live at the addresses. Find the name of the per-

son listed in the city directory for the address given by your patient as his or her home address on the initial patient registration or history form. If the person's name listed in the city directory is different than the patient's name, call the telephone company information operator and obtain the telephone number for the person listed in the city directory. Call the person listed at the patient's address and try to ascertain the patient's new address.

7. Search the city directory for the names and addresses of neighbors that live near the patient's given address. Obtain the telephone numbers of the neighbors and call them. A neighbor may be able to provide the patient's new address or a clue to the patient's whereabouts.
8. Major metropolitan areas have firms that specialize in tracing skipped debtors. Before employing the services of one of these firms, be sure your office confirms the fee arrangement. Try to arrange payment on the basis of a set fee contingent on finding the skipped patient. Avoid an arrangement based on an hourly fee for service. Payment by the hour may lead to a large expenditure of money with no results.
9. Check the name of the bank that the patient listed on his or her initial registration or history form. Call the bank and inquire whether the patient still has an active account. This may help confirm that the patient is still living in the area.
10. When tracing the skipped patient you must make sure you do not violate the Federal Fair Debt Collection Practices Act (United States Code title 15, sections 1692–1693). Some of the regulations related to acquiring information about a skipped patient include the following:

    a. When communicating with any person about the location of a patient, your office aide must identify him and state that he is confirming or correcting location information about the patient.
    b. Your office aide cannot state that the patient owes you a debt.

c. Your office aide cannot contact a person more than once seeking location information unless your aide reasonably believes that the earlier response of the person is erroneous or incomplete and that the person contacted now has correct or complete location information.
d. Your office may not use a postcard to communicate with any person regarding location information about a skipped patient.
e. Your office may not use any language or symbol on an envelope or telegram that indicates that the communication is related to the collection of a debt.

Claims Against a Bankrupt Patient

In common language, anyone who is financially "broke" is called bankrupt. Bankruptcy, however, is a specific legal entity and refers to a federal judicial procedure specifically detailed under title 11 of the United States Code (section 101-151326).

In a bankruptcy proceeding, a debtor comes into court and delivers property for liquidation and subsequent distribution to his or her creditors to a court-appointed officer (sometimes known as an *interim trustee*). The debtor thereby obtains a legal release from future liability for his or her debts and thus obtains a fresh economic start on life.

Although the bankruptcy proceedings are governed by federal laws, state laws may determine certain property rights related to matters such as who has rightful title to property, questions of marital status, and whether a debt exists, usuary interest has been charged, or the debtor is a partnership or corporation. State law may also establish what property may be claimed as exempt in a bankruptcy proceeding.

If your patient is the subject of a bankruptcy proceeding and owes a debt to you, you will be notified. Your notice will indicate whether there are assets available to satisfy your debt. If assets are available, you must file your proof of claim against the debtor in the United States Bankruptcy Court in your area.

Once you have been notified that a debtor has

declared bankruptcy, you must stop all of your usual collection procedures. The United States Code outlines the priority of debts to be paid by the trustee to creditors. Since professional fees are not based on any form of collateral (i.e., they lack a security interest), they are usually the last debts to be paid.

Your attorney should assist you with the preparation of your proof of claim and can answer specific questions related to bankruptcy proceedings.

Filing Claims Against the Estate of a Deceased Patient

If one of your patient's dies owing you professional fees, a claim may be made against the estate of the deceased patient. Every state has a legal procedure for the settlement of a deceased person's estate known as *probate*. Probate proceedings include granting letters of administration, collecting assets, allowing claims, paying debts, and distributing remaining property to the heirs as determined by the laws of descent or by the deceased's will.

To make a claim you should find out the name of the personal representative for the estate and send an itemized statement of the account by certified mail with a return receipt requested. The receipt will provide proof of the date that a claim was established against the estate. Almost all states have a statute of limitations designating a time period within which claims must be made against an estate.

The personal representative may accept or reject your claim (a so-called exception to your claim). If your claim is rejected, you will find it necessary to file a claim against the estate within the statute of limitations.

At the time that you send an itemized statement of the account to the personal representative of the estate, contact should be made with the appropriate court having jurisdiction over probate matters. The court having jurisdiction over matters of probate varies from state to state and even within states (see Appendix 28). Your office aide should request forms from the court handling probate matters for filing a claim against the estate of the deceased.

The following steps should be taken when a patient dies owing your office professional fees:

1. Send a bill to the surviving next of kin. Address the bill to The Estate of____(name of deceased patient).
2. Contact the court having jurisdiction over matters of probate. Inquire whether proceedings have been initiated.
3. Find out from the probate court who is responsible for handling distribution of the assets of the estate (the deceased's personal representative). If the deceased has a will, an executor will be appointed to handle and distribute the assets of the estate. The executor named in the will handles the disposition of the property. The executor is responsible for presenting the will, collecting the assets of the estate, and carrying out the final requests of the deceased as stated in the will along with paying the debts of the estate. In most jurisdictions, the executor is required to publish one or more legal notices in local newspapers notifying creditors to assert their claims. If the patient dies intestate (without a will), the court appoints an administrator to attend to the above details. See Appendix 28 for a list of courts having jurisdiction over the assets of an estate and the statute of limitations for filing a claim.
4. If the court indicates that no probate proceedings have been initiated, the inquiry should be repeated for several months thereafter, since it may take that long before heirs initiate legal proceedings. To obviate the need to inquire at frequent intervals, a legal instrument known as a *caveat* may be filed requesting that the probate court notify your office if probate proceedings are initiated at any time in the future. The court may charge a small fee for this service.
5. If probate proceedings have been initiated, your office should file your claim against the estate for professional fees. Have the court send you a claim form to file. Return the claim form by certified mail with a return receipt requested. Consult your attorney or the clerk of the court for specific legal details.

6. If a probate proceeding is not filed because there are insufficient assets in the estate to qualify for probate, or if the assets of the estate have passed directly to the heirs without necessity for probate proceedings to be filed, your office should send a bill for your professional fees to the personal representative of the estate by certified mail with a return receipt requested as proof that the claim was made. If there are no assets remaining in the deceased's estate, or if the assets have passed to heirs without necessity for probate, you may have no legal recourse for collecting your professional fees.
7. If a patient dies who is covered by Medicare insurance, the quickest way to receive payment of your professional fees is to file a claim with Medicare on an accept assignment basis. No signature is required of a family member or personal representative of the estate to submit this claim. A typed statement that the patient died on a specific date will substitute for the signature of the family or personal representative on the Medicare claim form HCFA-1490(2).
8. If you do not accept assignment, your bills for payment of your professional fees should be sent to the personal representative of the estate of the deceased as outlined above. The family members of the deceased, the personal representative of the estate, or other claimants have two options available to receive the deceased's Medicare Part B benefits when the physician does not accept assignment.

    a. The family member, personal representative, or other claimant may pay the physician's professional fees and then file for the Medicare reimbursement using claim HCFA-1660. This claim form may be obtained from the local Social Security Administration office.
    b. The family member, personal representative, or other claimant may file for the deceased's Medicare Part B benefits without first paying the physician's professional fees, but must submit the following documents to the Medicare intermediary:

(1) A signed statement that reads as follows: "I have assumed the legal obligation to pay (name of the physician) for services furnished to (name of the deceased Medicare beneficiary) on (date[s]). I hereby claim any Medicare benefits due for these services."
(2) A completed Medicare form HCFA-1490, which the claimant has signed in the space provided for the signature of the patient (line six of the HCFA-1490 form).
(3) A signed statement from the physician that signifies the physician refuses to accept assignment. This statement may take the form of a completed HCFA-1490 form that the physician has signed, indicating on line twelve this refusal to accept assignment.

The signed statement by the physician refusing to accept assignment is needed because the law requires that the physician be given the first opportunity to claim payment when the bill is unpaid. The physician may claim payment at any time before payment is made to a person who assumes the legal obligation to pay the bill. However, once payment is issued to such a person, the government has no further obligation with respect to the services involved, and the physician will therefore no longer qualify for payment.

A Final Note

Reading this book has been a step on the road to managing your practice. Although the dollar values quoted in this book may become outdated and the laws referred to may change, the concepts of organizing your practice for maximum efficiency and profit should remain constant and serve you well.

Good luck to you on the remainder of your journey.

Suggested Reading

Consumer Tell It To The Judge, Small Claims Courts and Consumer Complaints. Washington, D.C.: Department of Justice, 1980.

Current Opinions of the Judicial Council of the AMA, 1981. Monroe, Wis.: AMA, 1981.

Donoghue, W. E. *Complete Money Market Guide*. New York: Harper & Row, 1980.

Dorland's Illustrated Medical Dictionary (26th ed.). Philadelphia: Saunders, 1981.

Federal Tax Coordinator (2nd ed.). New York: The Research Institute of America, 1981.

Gorlick, S. *Now That You're Incorporated* (3rd ed.). Oradell, N.J.: Medical Economics, 1978.

Gorlick, S. (ed.). *The Whys and Wherefores of Corporate Practice*. Oradell, N.J.: Medical Economics, 1978.

Group Medical Practice in the U.S., 1975. Monroe, Wis.: AMA, 1975.

Group Practice Guidelines to Joining or Forming a Medical Group. Monroe, Wis.: AMA, 1981.

Hancock, W. A. *Executive's Guide to Business Law*. New York: McGraw-Hill, 1979.

Horty, J. *Hospital Law* (Looseleaf Service). Pittsburgh: Action Kit for Hospital Law, 1978.

Huffman, E. K. *Medical Record Management*. Berwyn, Ill.: Physicians' Record, 1972.

"Individual Retirement Plans." *Pension Plan Guide*. Issue #271, Part III. Chicago: Commerce Clearing House, April 11, 1980.

Klass, R. M. *The Physicians' Business Manual*. New York: Appleton-Century-Crofts, 1981.

Manual for Physicians. Jacksonville, Fla.: Blue Shield of Florida, 1980.

McCormick, J., Rushing, R., and Davis, W. G. *The Management of Medical Practice*. Cambridge, Mass.: Ballinger, 1978.

Physician Distribution and Medical Licensure in the U.S. Monroe, Wis.: AMA, 1979.

Planning Guide for Physicians' Medical Facilities. Monroe, Wis.: AMA, 1975.

Professional Corporations in Perspective. Monroe, Wis.: AMA, 1975.

Reference Guide to Policy and Official Statements. Monroe, Wis.: AMA, 1980.

Reschke, E. M. *The Medical Office: Organization and Management* (2nd ed.). New York: Harper & Row, 1980.

Rhodabarger, T. D. *Personal Money Management for Physicians*. Oradell, N.J.: Medical Economics, 1973.

Seld, L. G. *Harassment and Other Collection Taboos*. New York: National Association of Credit Managers, 1976.

Soukhandy, A. H. (ed.). *Webster's Medical Office Handbook*. Springfield, Mass.: Merriam, 1979.

"Tax Savings Plans for Self Employed." *Pension Plan Guide*. Issue #271, Part III. Chicago: Commerce Clearing House, April 11, 1980.
Warner, R. *Everybody's Guide to Small Claims Court*. Reading, Mass.: Addison-Wesley, 1980.
Wilson, J. *How to Get Paid for What You've Earned*. Oradell, N.J.: Medical Economics, 1974.
Ziegler, A. B. *Billing and Collections*. Oradell, N.J.: Medical Economics, 1979.
Ziegler, A. B. *Insurance and Third Party Payable Claims*. Oradell, N.J.: Medical Economics, 1979.
Concise Explanation of the Economic Recovery Tax Act of 1981. Englewood Cliffs, N.J.: Prentice-Hall, 1981.

Appendixes

The author has not investigated the organizations listed in these appendixes and assumes no responsibility for them.

Every effort has been made to insure the accuracy of the information contained in these appendixes. The author is not responsible for changes of address, clerical, or printer's errors.

Medical Groups in the U.S., 1975. Monroe, Wis.: AMA, 1975.

Physician Characteristics and Distribution in the U.S., 1981 Edition. Monroe, Wis.: AMA, 1981.

Physician Distribution and Medical Licensure in the U.S. Monroe, Wis.: AMA, 1979.

Profile of Medical Practice. Monroe, Wis.: AMA, 1981.

Socioeconomic Issues of Health. Monroe, Wis.: AMA, 1981.

Alabama
Medical Association of the State of Alabama
19 S. Jackson St.
P.O. Box 1900-C
Montgomery, AL 36197
205-263-6441

Alaska
Alaska State Medical Association
1135 W. Eighth Ave.
Suite 6
Anchorage, AK 99501
907-277-6891

Arizona
Arizona Medical Association, Inc.
810 W. Bethany Home Rd.
Phoenix, AZ 85013
602-246-8901

Arkansas
Arkansas Medical Society
214 N. Twelfth St.
Box 1208
Fort Smith, AR 72902
501-782-8218

California
California Medical Association
731 Market St.
San Francisco, CA 94103
415-777-2000

Colorado
Colorado Medical Society
1601 E. Nineteenth Ave.
Denver, CO 80218
303-861-1221

Connecticut
Connecticut State Medical Society
160 St. Ronan St.
New Haven, CT 06511
203-865-0587

Delaware
Medical Society of Delaware
1925 Lovering Ave.
Wilmington, DE 19806
302-658-7596

District of Columbia
Medical Society of District of Columbia
2007 Eye St., NW
Washington, DC 20006
202-223-2230

Florida
Florida Medical Association, Inc.
P.O. Box 2411
760 Riverside Ave.
Jacksonville, FL 32203
904-356-1571

Georgia
Medical Association of Georgia
938 Peachtree St., NE
Atlanta, GA 30309
404-876-7535

Hawaii
Hawaii Medical Association
320 Ward Ave., Suite 200
Honolulu, HI 96814
808-536-7702

Idaho
Idaho Medical Association
P.O. Box 2668
407 W. Bannock St.
Boise, ID 83701
208-344-7888

Illinois
Illinois State Medical Society
55 E. Monroe
Suite 3510
Chicago, IL 60603
312-782-1654

Indiana
Indiana State Medical Association
3935 N. Meridian
Indianapolis, IN 46208
317-925-7545

Iowa
Iowa Medical Society
1001 Grand Ave.
West Des Moines, IA 50265
515-223-1401

Kansas
Kansas Medical Society
1300 Topeka Blvd.
Topeka, KS 66612
913-235-2383

Kentucky
Kentucky Medical Association
3532 Ephraim McDowell Dr.
Louisville, KY 40205
502-459-9790

Louisiana
Louisiana State Medical Society
1700 Josephine St.
New Orleans, LA 70113
504-561-1033

Maine
Maine Medical Association
524 Western Ave.
Augusta, ME 04330
203-622-3374

Maryland
Medical & Chirurgical Faculty of Maryland
1211 Cathedral St.
Baltimore, MD 21201
301-539-0872

Massachusetts
Massachusetts Medical Society
22 Fenway
Boston, MA 02215
617-536-8812

Michigan
Michigan State Medical Society
P.O. Box 950
120 W. Saginaw
East Lansing, MI 48823
517-337-1351

Minnesota
Minnesota Medical Association
Health Associations Center
2221 University Ave., SE
Suite 400
Minneapolis, MN 55414
612-378-1875

Mississippi
Mississippi State Medical Association
735 Riverside Dr.
P.O. Box 5229
Jackson, MS 39216
601-354-5433

Missouri
Missouri State Medical Association
P.O. Box 1028
113 Madison St.
Jefferson City, MO 65101
314-636-5151

Montana
Montana Medical Association
2021 Eleventh Ave.
Suite 12
Helena, MT 59601
406-443-4000

Nebraska
Nebraska Medical Association
1512 First National Bank Bldg.
Lincoln, NE 68508
402-432-7585

Nevada
Nevada State Medical Association
3660 Baker Ln.
Reno, NV 89509
702-825-6788

New Hampshire
New Hampshire Medical Society
4 Park St.
Concord, NH 03301
603-224-1909

New Jersey
Medical Society of New Jersey
2 Princess Rd.
Lawrenceville, NJ 08648
609-896-1766

New Mexico
New Mexico Medical Society
P.O. Box 9366
2650 Yale Blvd., SE
Albuquerque, NM 87106
505-247-0539

New York
Medical Society of the State of New York
420 Lakeville Rd.
Lake Success, NY 11040
516-488-6100

North Carolina
North Carolina Medical Society
222 N. Person St.
P.O. Box 27167
Raleigh, NC 27611
919-833-3836

North Dakota
North Dakota Medical Association
P.O. Box 1198
810 E. Roffer Ave.
Bismarck, ND 58501
701-223-9475

Ohio
Ohio State Medical Association
600 S. High St.
Columbus, OH 43215
614-228-6971

Oklahoma
Oklahoma State Medical Association
601 NW Expressway
Oklahoma City, OK 73118
405-843-9571

Oregon
Oregon Medical Association
5210 Corbett St., SW
Portland, OR 97201
503-226-1555

Pennsylvania
Pennsylvania Medical Society
P.O. Box 301
20 Erford Rd.
Lemoyne, PA 17043
717-763-7151

Rhode Island
Rhode Island Medical Society
Providence Medical Association
106 Francis St.
Providence, RI 02903
401-331-3207

South Carolina
South Carolina Medical Association
3325 Medical Park Rd.
Box 11188
Columbia, SC 29211
803-252-6311

South Dakota
South Dakota State Medical Association
608 West Ave., North
Sioux Falls, SD 57104
605-336-1965

Tennessee
Tennessee Medical Association
112 Louise Ave.
Nashville, TN 37203
615-327-1451

Texas
Texas Medical Association
1801 N. Lamar Blvd.
Austin, TX 78701
512-447-6704

Utah
Utah State Medical Association
540 Fifth St. South
Salt Lake City, UT 84102
801-355-7477

Vermont
Vermont State Medical Society
136 Main St.
Montpelier, VT 05602
802-223-7898

Virginia
Medical Society of Virginia
4205 Dover Rd.
Richmond, VA 23221
804-353-2721

Washington
Washington State Medical Association
2033 Sixth Ave.
Seattle, WA 98121
206-623-4801

West Virginia
West Virginia State Medical Association
Charleston National Plaza
P.O. Box 1031
Charleston, WV 25324
304-346-0551

Wisconsin
State Medical Society of Wisconsin
330 E. Lakeside St.
Box 1109
Madison, WI 53701
608-257-6781

Wyoming
Wyoming Medical Society
1920 Evans St.
P.O. Drawer 4009
Cheyenne, WY 82001
307-635-2424

Appendix 3. A Selection of National Medical Specialty Societies with Placement Services

American Academy of Dermatology
820 Davis St.
Evanston, IL 60201
Attention: Placement Service

The American Academy of Family Physicians
1740 W. Ninety-second St.
Kansas City, MO 64114

American Academy of Neurology
4015 W. Sixty-fifth St.
Suite 302
Minneapolis, MN 55435
Attention: Placement Service

American Academy of Ophthalmology
P.O. Box 7424
1833 Fillmore St.
San Francisco, CA 94120
Attention: Ophthalmology Placement Exchange

American Academy of Orthopedic Surgeons
444 N. Michigan Ave.
Chicago, IL 60611
Attention: Placement Bureau

American Academy of Otolaryngology—Head and Neck Surgery
15 Second St., SW
Rochester, MN 55901
Attention: Placement Bureau

American Academy of Pediatrics
1801 Hinman Ave.
Evanston, IL 60204
Attention: Placement Service

American College of Emergency Physicians
P.O. Box 61911
Dallas, TX 75261
Attention: Placement Service

American College of Radiology
20 N. Wacker Dr.
Chicago, IL 60606
Attention: Professional Bureau

The American Council of Otolaryngology
1100 Seventeenth St., NW
Suite 602
Washington, DC 20036
Attention: Job Information Exchange Service

American Psychiatric Association
1700 Eighteenth St., NW
Washington, DC 20009
Attention: Placement Service

American Society of Anesthesiologists
515 Busse Highway
Parkridge, IL 60068
Attention: Placement Service

College of American Pathologists
7400 N. Skokie Blvd.
Skokie, IL 60077
Attention: Placement Bureau

The Society of Nuclear Medicine
475 Park Ave., South
New York, NY 10016
Attention: Placement Coordinator

Appendix 4. A Selection of State and Federal Organizations with Physician Recruitment Services

Appalachia Health Professions Clearinghouse
8294 C Old Courthouse Rd.
Vienna, VA 22180

Central Intelligence Agency
Dept. A, Room 821-AM
P.O. Box 1925
Washington, DC 20013
Attention: Office of Medical Services

Health Services Consortium
925 Seneca St.
P.O. Box 1930
Seattle, WA 98111
Attention: Physician Recruiter

Indian Health Service
California Program Office
2800 Cottage Way, #E-1831
Sacramento, CA 95825
Attention: Chief Medical Officer

New Physician for Wisconsin
Office of Rural Health–University of Wisconsin
777 S. Mills
Madison, WI 53715

North Carolina Office of Rural Health Services
P.O. Box 12200-M
Raleigh, NC 27605
Attention: Physician Recruitment Coordinator

North Central Pennsylvania Regional Planning and Development Commission
122 Center St.
Box 377
Ridgway, PA 15853
Attention: Deputy Director, Development

State of Illinois
Executive Recruitment Division
205 W. Wacker Dr.
Suite 1900
Chicago, IL 60606
Attention: Executive Recruitment Representative

Virginia Council on Health and Medical Care, Inc.
100 E. Franklin St.
Richmond, VA 23219
Attention: Director

Appendix 5. A Selection of Universities and Medical Schools with Physician Recruitment Services

Network of Rural Health Programs
University of Utah Medical Center
50 N. Medical Dr.
Salt Lake City, UT 84132
Attention: Coordinator of Recruitment

Office of Rural Health
University of North Dakota
School of Medicine
501 Columbia Rd.
Grand Forks, ND 58202
Attention: Program Assistant

Southern Illinois University
School of Medicine
Office of Health Systems Research
Practice Opportunity Program
P.O. Box 3926
Springfield, IL 62708

University of Alabama
College of Community Health Sciences
P.O. Box 6291
University, AL 35486

University of Wisconsin
New Physicians for Wisconsin
Office of Rural Health
Department of Family Medicine and Practice
777 S. Mills
Madison, WI 53715

Appendix 6. A Selection of Health Maintenance Organizations with Physician Recruitment Services

Anchor
Organization for Health Maintenance
600 S. Paulina
764 Academic Facility
Chicago, IL 60612

East Nassau Medical Group
350 S. Broadway
Hicksville, NY 11801
Attention: Administration

Group Health Service
4200 Fashion Square Blvd.
Saginaw, MI 48603
Attention: Medical Director

Health Care Plan Medical Center
120 Gardenville Pkwy., West
West Seneca, NY 14224

Northwest Permanente, P.C.
1500 SW First Ave.
11th Floor
Portland, OR 97201

Ohio Permanente Medical Group
2475 East Blvd.
Cleveland, OH 44120

Permanente Medical Group
5755 Cottle Rd.
San Jose, CA 95123

Prime Health
6801 E. 117th St.
Kansas City, MO 64134
Attention: Medical Director

Quad-City Health Plan
2435 Kimberly Rd.
Bettendorf, IA 52728
Attention: Executive Director

Southern California Permanente Medical Group
4747 Sunset Blvd. #B-80
Los Angeles, CA 90027
Attention: Physician Placement

Appendix 7. A Selection of Group Practices with Physician Placement Services

American Group Practice Association
Group Practice Placement Service
20 S. Quaker Ln.
Alexandria, VA 22314
Attention: Director, Placement Service

Hygeia Facilities Foundation, Inc.
Box 217
Whitesville, WV 25209
Attention: Administrator

Medical Treatment Centers, Inc.
8200 E. Sunrise Blvd.
Plantation, FL 33322
Attention: Professional Services

Neighborhood Medical
309 Civic Center Dr. West
Santa Anna, CA 92201
Attention: Administrator

The Wheeling Clinic
Wheeling, WV 26003
Attention: Recruitment Chairman

Appendix 8. A Selection of Hospital and Clinic Management Companies with Physician Recruitment or Placement Services

Advanced Health Systems, Inc.
2415 S. 2300 West
Salt Lake City, UT 84119
Attention: Physician Recruitment Coordinator

American Medical International
6400 Powers Ferry Rd.
Atlanta, GA 30339
Attention: Physician Relations

A. E. Brim & Associates
177 NE 102nd Ave.
Portland, OR 97236
Attention: Consultant Physician Services

Calumet Memorial Hospital
614 Memorial Dr.
Chilton, WI 53014
Attention: Administrator

Carolinas Hospital and Health Services
P.O. Box 12546
Raleigh, NC 27605
Attention: Community Development Coordinator

Family Health Care Centers
444 N. Michigan Ave.
Suite 3650
Chicago, IL 60611
Attention: President

Hospital Affiliates International
Western Division
7616 L.B.J. Freeway, S-303
Dallas, TX 75251
Attention: Physician Relations

Hospital Affiliates Management Corp.
Eastern Division
6520 Powers Ferry Rd., S-300
Atlanta, GA 30339
Attention: Physician Relations

Hospital Affiliates Management Corp.
Western Division
6225 U.S. Highway 290 E.
Suite 201
Austin, TX 78723

Hospital Corporation of America
P.O. Box 550
1 Park Plaza
Nashville, TN 37202
Attention: Physician Recruitment

Hospital Management Associates
2180 W. First St.
Suite 510
Fort Myers, FL 33901
Attention: Physician Recruitment

Humana Corp.
P.O. Box 1430
Louisville, KY 40201
Attention: Professional Relations

Jackson & Coker
4488 N. Shallowford Rd.
Suite 1040
Atlanta, GA 30338
Attention: President

National Medical Enterprises, Inc.
11620 Wilshire Blvd.
Los Angeles, CA 90025
Attention: Physician Relations

Qualicare
P.O. Box 24189
New Orleans, LA 70184
Attention: Director of
Physician Recruiting

St. Mary's Hospital
1800 E. Lakeshore Dr.
Decatur, IL 62525
Attention: Medical
Director

The Woodward Group
35 E. Wacker Dr.
Suite 3400
Chicago, IL 60601
Attention: President,
Executive Search
Division

Gary S. Bell Associates, Inc.
393 Crescent Ave.
Wyckoff, NJ 07481

Blendow, Crowley & Oliver
185 Front St.
Suite 205
Danville, CA 94526

Bryant Bureau
1040 Bayview Dr.
Suite 201
Ft. Lauderdale, FL 33304
Attention: Medical Director

John Conway Associates
2040 W. Wisconsin Ave.
Milwaukee, WI 53233
Attention: Search Division

The Corson Group
515 Madison Ave.
New York, NY 10022

Durham Medical Search
268 Main St.
Suite 600
Buffalo, NY 14202

Fox Hill Associates
W156 N8327 Pilgrim Rd.
Menomonee Falls, WI 53051

H. S. Placement Service, Inc.
1345 W. Mason
P.O. Box 3247
Green Bay, WI 54303
Attention: Director, Medical Division

Health Resources Corp.
201 Evans Rd.
Suite 414
New Orleans, LA 70123
Attention: Physician Representative

Health Resources, Ltd.
River Road Professional Bldg.
Box 12220
Kansas City, MO 64152

Jonas & Associates, Inc.
3333 N. Mayfair Rd.
Suite 313
Milwaukee, WI 53222
Attention: Medical Director

Management Recruiters
15 Bank St.
Suite 204
Stamford, CT 06901
Attention: Physician Recruiter

Management Recruiters
Twin Tower N.
Suite 535
8585 N. Stemmons Freeway
Dallas, TX 75075
Attention: Physician Recruiter

Management Recruiters–Evansville
Riverside One
101 Court St.
Suite 209
Evansville, IN 47708
Attention: Medical Recruiter

Marsh/Bennett Associates, Inc.
2741 N. Twenty-ninth Ave., #212
Hollywood, FL 33020
Attention: Director, Medical Placement

Medi-Search
1800 M St., NW
Suite 310 North
Washington, DC 20036

Medical Development Concepts, Inc.
10500 Clara Dr.
Suite A-1
Roswell, GA 30076

Medical Resources, Inc.
38 Frazier Ave.
Suite A
Chattanooga, TN 37405

Medical Search Associates
18550 Gilmore St.
Reseda, CA 91335
Attention: Medical
Director

Medical Search Division,
M.R.I.
104-70 Queens Blvd.
Suite 301
Forest Hills, NY 11375
Attention: Physician
Recruiters

Meridian/Medical
25 W. Forty-third St.
New York, NY 10036
Attention: Physician
Recruitment

Mitchell & Associates
P.O. Box 4296
Yuma, AZ 85364
Attention: Physician
Recruiting Division

The C. B. Mueller Co., Inc.
550 E. Fourth St.
Cincinnati, OH 45202

National Medical
Placement Services, Inc.
P.O. Box 156-J
Tiburon, CA 94920

Nationwide Health Search
6717 Evergreen Canyon Rd.
Suite 777
Oklahoma City, OK 73132

Earle Nicklas, Inc.
Box 711
Cooperstown, NY 13326

Norton-Children's
Hospitals, Inc.
Division of Planning and
Management
224 E. Broadway
Louisville, KY 40202

Physician Search
Consultants, Inc.
9502 B Lee Highway
Fairfax, VA 22031
Attention: Director,
Physician Placement

Professional Management
Group, Inc.
4330 Medical Dr.
Suite 500
San Antonio, TX 78229

Professional Practice
Management
1102 Kingswood Dr.
Humble, TX 77339

Sisters of St. Joseph
Coordinated Services
3720 E. Bayley
Wichita, KS 67218
Attention: Medical
Personnel Recruitment
Coordinator

M. C. Staachak, M.D.,
& Associates
Manor Bldg., Fifth Floor
Pittsburgh, PA 15219

VIP Physician Practice
Development Network
80 S. Lake Ave.
Suite 820
Pasadena, CA 91101

Whittaker Health
Resources
2942 N. Twenty-fourth St.
Suite 216
Phoenix, AZ 85016

The Woodward Group, Inc.
35 E. Wacker Dr.
Suite 3400
Chicago, IL 60601

Roth Young of Seattle
515 116th NE
Suite 250
Bellevue, WA 98004

Appendix 10. Consultants to Organizations for Physician Recruitment

American Physician Association
6419 Independence Ave.
Woodland Hills, CA 91367

Bryant Bureau
Medical Services Division
1605 Lamy Ln.
Suite B
Monroe, LA 71202

The Corson Group, Inc.
515 Madison Ave.
New York, NY 10022

Dorothea Bowlby
30 N. Michigan Ave.
Suite 405
Chicago, IL 60602

Earle Nicklas, Inc.
Box 711
Cooperstown, NY 13326

Envision
Publishers of *Physicians 1981*
3429 Flintridge Dr.
Lexington, KY 40502

Manpower Development
NKI, Inc.
224 E. Broadway
Louisville, KY 40202

Professional Management Group, Inc.
4330 Medical Dr.
Suite 500
San Antonio, TX 78229

Prudential Health Care Plan, Inc.
213 Washington St.
Suite A
Newark, NJ 07101

Saffer
505 Fifth Ave.
New York, NY 10017

Sampson, Neill & Wilkins, Inc.
543 Valley Rd.
Upper Montclair, NJ 07043

Worldwide Health Consultants, Inc.
1271 Avenue of the Americas
New York, NY 10020

Appendix 11. A Selection of Emergency Medical Recruitment Services

Emergency Consultants, Inc.
2240 S. Airport Rd.
Traverse City, MI 49684

Emergency Medical Services Associates
8200 N. Sunrise Blvd.
Plantation, FL 33322

National Emergency Services, Inc.
P.O. Box 156
Tiburon, CA 94920

National Emergency Services, Inc.
4419 Cowan Rd.
Tucker, GA 30084

National Emergency Services, Inc.
9953 Lewis & Clark
St. Louis, MO 63136

National Emergency Services, Inc.
1 Hollow Lane
Lake Success, NY 11042

National Emergency Services, Inc.
1955 S. Reynolds
Toledo, OH 43614

National Emergency Services, Inc.
3301 Airport Freeway
Bedford, TX 76021

NEEMA Emergency Medical
399 Market St.
Suite 400
Philadelphia, PA 19106

Spectrum Emergency Care, Inc.
970 Executive Pkwy.
St. Louis, MO 63141

Appendix 12. Other Placement Organizations

Alabama Hospital
Association
P.O. Box 17059
East Station
Montgomery, AL 36193

Correctional Medical
Systems
970 Executive Pkwy.
St. Louis, MO 63141

Joint Commission on
Accreditation of
Hospitals
875 N. Michigan Ave.
Chicago, IL 60611

Locum Tenens Group, Inc.
2301 Bellevue Ave., 4-W.
Los Angeles, CA 90026

Medical Center, Ltd.
P.O. Box 309
131 New London Turnpike
Glastonbury, CT 06033

Pharmaceutical Industry
Placement Service
19 Berkeley Pl.
Montclair, NJ 07042

Architectual Services
American Institute of Architects
1735 New York Ave., NW
Washington, DC 20006

Ellerbe, Inc.
1 Appletree Sq.
Bloomington, MN 55420

Harold J. Westin and Associates, Inc.
45 E. Eighth St.
St. Paul, MN 55101

Marshall Erdman and Associates, Inc.
5117 University Ave.
Madison, WI 53705

Medical Construction Management Corp.
5201 Old Middleton Rd.
Madison, WI 53705

Nationwide Medical-Dental Bldg. Corp.
797 Market St.
Oregon, WI 53575

Professional Office Bldg., Inc.
Doctors Park
Madison, WI 53705

Alabama State Board of Medical Examiners
P.O. Box 946
Montgomery, AL 36102

Alaska State Medical Board
Department of Occupational Licensing
Pouch D
Juneau, AK 99811

Arizona State Board of Medical Examiners
5060-N Nineteenth Ave.
3rd Floor West
Phoenix, AZ 85015

Arkansas State Medical Board
P.O. Box 102
Harrisburg, AR 72432

California Board of Medical Quality Assurance
1430 Howe Ave.
Sacramento, CA 95825

Colorado Board of Medical Examiners
132 State Services Bldg.
1525 Sherman St.
Denver, CO 80203

Connecticut Medical Examining Board
79 Elm St.
Hartford, CT 06115

Delaware Board of Medical Practice
Margaret M. O'Neill Bldg.
Third Floor
Dover, DE 19901

District of Columbia Commission on Licensure to Practice the Healing Arts
614 H St., NW
Room 114
Washington, DC 20001

Florida Board of Medical Examiners
130 N. Monroe St.
Tallahassee, FL 32301

Georgia Composite Board of Medical Examiners
166 Pryor St., SW
Atlanta, GA 30303

Hawaii Board of Medical Examiners
Department of Regulatory Agencies
P.O. Box 541
Honolulu, HI 96809

Idaho State Board of Medicine
700 W. State
Boise, ID 83707

Illinois Department of Registration and Education
320 W. Washington St.
Springfield, IL 62786

Indiana Medical Licensing Board
700 N. High School Rd.
Suite 201
Indianapolis, IN 46224

Iowa State Board of Medical Examiners
State Capitol Complex
Executive Hills West
Des Moines, IA 50319

Kansas State Board of Healing Arts
503 Kansas Ave.
Topeka, KS 66603

Kentucky State Board of Healing Arts
3532 Ephraim McDowell Dr.
Louisville, KY 40205

Louisiana State Board of Medical Examiners
830 Union St.
Suite 100
New Orleans, LA 70112

Maine State Board of Registration in Medicine
100 College Ave.
Waterville, ME 04901

Maryland Board of Medical Examiners
201 W. Preston St.
Fifth Floor
Baltimore, MD 21201

Massachusetts Board of Registration in Medicine
Leverett Saltonstall Bldg.
100 Cambridge St.
Room 1511
Boston, MA 02202

Michigan Board of Medicine
P.O. Box 30018
Lansing, MI 48909

Minnesota State Board of Medical Examiners
Suite 352
717 Delaware St., SE
Minneapolis, MN 55414

Mississippi State Board of Medical Licensure
P.O. Box 1700
Jackson, MS 39205

Missouri State Board of Registration for the Healing Arts
P.O. Box 4
Jefferson City, MO 65102

Montana State Board of Medical Examiners
Lalonde Bldg.
Helena, MT 59601

Nebraska State Board of Examiners in Medicine and Surgery
P.O. Box 95007
Lincoln, NE 68508

Nevada State Board of Medical Examiners
P.O. Box 7238
Reno, NV 89510

New Hampshire State Board of Registration in Medicine
Health and Welfare Building
Hazen Dr.
Concord, NH 03301

New Jersey State Board of Medical Examiners
28 W. State St.
Trenton, NJ 08608

New Mexico State Board of Medical Examiners
227 E. Palace Ave.
Suite "O"
Santa Fe, NM 87501

New York Board of Medicine
Division of Professional Licensing
Cultural Education Center
Empire State Plaza
Room 3029
Albany, NY 12230

North Carolina State Board of Medical Examiners
222 N. Person St.
Suite 214
Raleigh, NC 27601

North Dakota Board of Medical Examiners
418 E. Rosser Ave.
Bismarck, ND 58501

Ohio State Medical Board
65 S. Front St., #510
Columbus, OH 43215

Oklahoma State Board of Medical Examiners
P.O. Box 18256
Oklahoma City, OK 73154

Oregon Board of Medical Examiners
1002 Loyalty Bldg.
317 SW Alder St.
Portland, OR 97204

Pennsylvania State Board of Medical Education and Licensure
P.O. Box 2649
Harrisburg, PA 17120

Rhode Island State Department of Health
104 Cannon Bldg.
75 Davis St.
Providence, RI 02903

South Carolina State Board
of Medical Examiners
1315 Blanding St.
Columbia, SC 29201

South Dakota State Board
of Medical and
Osteopathic Examiners
608 West Ave., North
Sioux Falls, SD 57104

Tennessee State Board of
Medical Examiners
320 R. S. Gass State Office
Bldg.
Ben Allen Rd.
Nashville, TN 37216

Texas State Board of
Medical Examiners
211 E. Seventh St., #900
Austin, TX 78701

Utah Department of
Registration
330 E. Fourth St., South
Salt Lake City, UT 84111

Vermont State Board of
Medical Practice
Administration Post Office
13 Baldwin St.
Montpelier, VT 05602

Virginia State Board of
Medicine
Seaboard Bldg.
3600 W. Broad St.
Room 453
Richmond, VA 23230

Washington Professional
Licensing Division
P.O. Box 9649
Olympia, WA 98504

West Virginia Board of
Medicine
State Office Bldg.
1800 Washington St.
Charleston, WV 25305

Wisconsin Medical
Examining Board
1400 E. Washington Ave.
Madison, WI 53702

Wyoming Board of Medical
Examiners
Hathaway Bldg.
Fourth Floor
Cheyenne, WY 82002

Alabama
Medicare-BlueCross/Blue Shield of Alabama
P.O. Box C-140
Birmingham, AL 35205

Alaska
Medicare-Aetna Life & Casualty (For Alaska)
1500 SW First Ave.
Portland, OR 97201

Arizona
Medicare-Aetna Life & Casualty
3010 W. Fairmont Ave.
Phoenix, AZ 85017

Arkansas
Medicare-Arkansas Blue Cross/Blue Shield
P.O. Box 1418
Little Rock, AR 72203

California
Medicare-Occidental Life Insurance Company of California
P.O. Box 54904, Terminal Annex
Los Angeles, CA 90054
All counties south of and including San Luis Obispo

Medicare-Blue Shield of California
P.O. Box 7968, Rincon Annex
San Francisco, CA 94120
Counties north of San Luis Obispo

Colorado
Medicare-Colorado Medical Services, Inc.
700 Broadway
Denver, CO 80273

Connecticut
Medicare-Connecticut General Life Insurance Company
200 Pratt St.
Meriden, CT 06450

Delaware
Medicare-Blue Cross/Blue Shield of Delaware
201 W. Fourteenth St.
Wilmington, DE 19899

District of Columbia
Medicare-Medical Service of D. C.
550 Twelfth St. SW
Washington, DC 20024

Florida
Medicare-Blue Shield of Florida, Inc.
P.O. Box 2525
Jacksonville, FL 32231
All counties except Dade and Monroe

Medicare-Group Health Insurance
P.O. Box 341370
Miami, FL 33134
Dade and Monroe counties

Georgia
Medicare-The Prudential Insurance Company of America
P.O. Box 95466
Executive Park Station
Atlanta, GA 30347

Hawaii
Medicare-Aetna Life & Casualty
P.O. Box 3947
Honolulu, HI 96812

Idaho
Medicare-The Equitable Life Assurance Society
P.O. Box 8048
Boise, ID 83707

Illinois
Medicare-E.D.S. Federal Corp.
Medicare Claims
P.O. Box 66906
Chicago, IL 60666

Indiana
Medicare-Part B
120 W. Market St.
Indianapolis, IN 46201

Iowa
Medicare-Iowa Medical Service
636 Grand Ave.
Des Moines, IA 50307

Kansas
Medicare-Blue Shield of Kansas City
P.O. Box 169
Kansas City, MO 64141
Johnson and Wyandotte counties, Kansas

Medicare-Kansas Blue Shield
P.O. Box 239
Topeka, KS 66601
Except Johnson and Wyandotte counties, Kansas

Kentucky
Medicare-Metropolitan Life Insurance Company
1218 Harrodsburg Rd.
Lexington, KY 40504

Louisiana
Medicare-Pan-American Life Insurance Company
P.O. Box 60450
New Orleans, LA 70160

Maine
Medicare-Blue Shield of Massachusetts-Maine Claims
P.O. Box 2410
Boston, MA 02208

Maryland
Medicare
550 Twelfth St., SW
Washington, DC 20024
Montgomery and Prince George counties

Medicare-Maryland Blue Shield, Inc.
700 E. Joppa Rd.
Towson, MD 21204
Except Montgomery and Prince George counties

Massachusetts
Medicare-Blue Shield of Massachusetts, Inc.
P.O. Box 2194
Boston, MA 02106

Michigan
Medicare-Blue Shield of Michigan
P.O. Box 2201
Detroit, MI 48231

Minnesota
Medicare-The Travelers Insurance Company
8120 Penn Ave., South
Bloomington, MN 55431
Anoka, Dakota, Filmore, Goodhue, Hennepin, Houston, Olmstead, Ramsey, Wabasha, Washington, and Winona counties

Medicare-Blue Shield of Minnesota
P.O. Box 43357
Minneapolis, MN 55164
Except counties listed for preceding address

Mississippi
Medicare-The Travelers Insurance Company
P.O. Box 22545
Jackson, MS 39205

Missouri
Medicare-Blue Shield of Kansas City
P.O. Box 169
Kansas City, MO 64141
Andrew, Atchison, Bates, Benton, Buchanon, Caldwell, Carroll, Cass, Clinton, Davies, DeKalb, Gentry, Grundy, Harrison, Henry, Holt, Jackson, Johnson, Lafayette, Livingston, Mercer, Nodaway, Pettis, Platte, Ray, St. Clair, Saline, Vernon, and Worth counties

Medicare-General
American Life Insurance
Company
P.O. Box 505
St. Louis, MO 63166

Montana
Medicare-Montana
Physicians' Service
P.O. Box 4310
Helena, MT 59601

Nebraska
Medicare-Mutual of
Omaha Insurance
Company
P.O. Box 456
Downtown Station
Omaha, NE 68101

Nevada
Medicare-Aetna Life &
Casualty
4600 Kietzke Land
P.O. Box 7290
Reno, NV 89510

New Hampshire
Medicare-New Hampshire-
Vermont Physician
Service
2 Pillsbury St.
Concord, NH 03301

New Jersey
Medicare-The Prudential
Insurance Company of
America
P.O. Box 3000
Linwood, NJ 08221

New Mexico
Medicare-The Equitable
Life Assurance Society
P.O. Box 3070, Station D
Albuquerque, NM 87110

New York
Medicare-Blue Cross/Blue
Shield of Greater New
York
P.O. Box 458, Murray Hill
Station
New York, NY 10016
Bronx, Columbia,
Delaware, Dutchess,
Greene, Kings, Nassau,
New York, Orange,
Putnam, Richmond,
Rockland, Suffolk,
Sullivan, Ulster, and
Westchester counties

Medicare-Group Health,
Inc.
P.O. Box A966
Times Square Station
New York, NY 10036
Queens county

Medicare-Blue Shield of
Western New York
P.O. Box 600
Binghamton, NY 13902
All other counties except
those listed for
preceding two addresses

North Carolina
Medicare-Prudential
Insurance Company of
America
P.O. Box 2126
High Point, NC 27261

North Dakota
Medicare-Blue Shield of
North Dakota
301 Eighth St., South
Fargo, ND 58102

Ohio
Medicare-Nationwide
Mutual Insurance
Company
P.O. Box 47
Columbus, OH 43216

Oklahoma
Medicare-Aetna Life &
Casualty
Jamestown Office Park
3031 NW Sixty-fourth St.
Oklahoma City, OK 73116

Oregon
Medicare-Aetna Life & Casualty
1500 SW First Ave.
Portland, OR 97201

Pennsylvania
Medicare-Pennsylvania Blue Shield
Blue Shield Bldg.
Box 65
Camp Hill, PA 17011

Rhode Island
Medicare-Blue Shield of Rhode Island
444 Westminster Mall
Providence, RI 02901

South Carolina
Medicare-Blue Shield of South Carolina
Drawer F
Forest Acres Branch
Columbia, SC 29260

South Dakota
Medicare-South Dakota Medical Service, Inc.
160 W. Madison
Sioux Falls, SD 57104

Tennessee
Medicare-The Equitable Life Assurance Society
P.O. Box 1465
Nashville, TN 37202

Texas
Medicare-Group Medical and Surgical Service
P.O. Box 222147
Dallas, TX 75222

Utah
Medicare-Blue Shield of Utah
P.O. Box 30270
2455 Parley's Way
Salt Lake City, UT 84125

Vermont
Medicare-New Hampshire-Vermont Physician Service
2 Pillsbury St.
Concord, NH 03301

Virginia
Medicare
550 Twelfth St., SW
Washington, DC 20024
Arlington and Fairfax counties, Virginia; cities of Alexandria, Fallschurch, and Fairfax

Medicare-The Travelers Insurance Company
P.O. Box 26463
Richmond, VA 23261
All counties except those listed for preceding address

Washington
Medicare-Washington Physicians' Service
Fourth and Battery Bldg.
Sixth Floor
2401 Fourth Ave.
Seattle, WA 98121

West Virginia
Medicare of West Virginia
Nationwide Mutual Insurance Company
P.O. Box 57
Columbus, OH 43216

Wisconsin
Medicare-Surgical Care–Blue Shield
P.O. Box 2049
Milwaukee, WI 53201
Milwaukee county

Medicare-Wisconsin Physicians' Service
P.O. Box 1787
Madison, WI 53701
Except Milwaukee county

Wyoming
Medicare-The Equitable Life Assurance Society
P.O. Box 628
Cheyenne, WY 82001

Alabama
Blue Cross and Blue Shield of Alabama
P.O. Box 995
450 Riverchase Pkwy.
Birmingham, AL 35298

Alaska
See Blue Cross of Washington and Alaska

Arizona
Blue Cross and Blue Shield of Arizona, Inc.
P.O. Box 13466
321 W. Indian School Rd.
Phoenix, AZ 85013

Arkansas
Arkansas Blue Cross and Blue Shield, Inc.
P.O. Box 2181
601 Gaines St.
Little Rock, AR 72203

California
Blue Shield of California
P.O. Box 3637
2 N. Point
San Francisco, CA 94119

Blue Cross of Southern California
P.O. Box 70000
21555 Oxnard St.
Van Nuys, CA 91470

Blue Cross of Northern California
1950 Franklin St.
Oakland, CA 94659

Colorado
Blue Cross and Blue Shield of Colorado
700 Broadway
Denver, CO 80273

Connecticut
Blue Cross and Blue Shield of Connecticut, Inc.
P.O. Box 504
370 Bassett Rd.
North Haven, CT 06473

Delaware
Blue Cross and Blue Shield of Delaware, Inc.
P.O. Box 1991
201 W. Fourteenth St.
Wilmington, DE 19801

District of Columbia
District of Columbia-Group Hospital, Inc.
550 Twelfth St., SW
Washington, DC 20024

Florida
Blue Cross and Blue Shield of Florida, Inc.
P.O. Box 1798
532 Riverside Ave.
Jacksonville, FL 32231

Georgia
Blue Cross and Blue Shield of Georgia/Atlanta, Inc.
P.O. Box 4445
Atlanta, GA 30302

Blue Cross of Georgia/Columbus, Inc.
P.O. Box 7368
2357 Warm Springs Rd.
Columbus, GA 31904

Hawaii
Hawaii Medical Service Association
P.O. Box 860
1504 Kapiolani Blvd.
Honolulu, HI 96814

Idaho
Blue Cross of Idaho Health Service, Inc.
P.O. Box 7408
1501 Federal Way
Boise, ID 83705

Blue Shield of Idaho
P.O. Box 1106
1602 Twenty-first Ave.
Lewiston, ID 83501

Illinois
Health Care Service Corp.
P.O. Box 1364
233 N. Michigan Ave.
Chicago, IL 60690

Rockford Blue Cross
(Illinois Hospital and
Health Service, Inc.)
227 Wyman St.
Rockford, IL 61101

Indiana
Blue Cross of Indiana
120 W. Market St.
Indianapolis, IN 46204

Blue Shield of Indiana
120 W. Market St.
Indianapolis, IN 46204

Iowa
Blue Cross and Blue Shield
of Iowa
636 Grand Ave.
Des Moines, IA 50307

Blue Cross of Western
Iowa and South Dakota
P.O. Box 1677
Hamilton Blvd. and I-29
Sioux City, IA 51102

Kansas
Blue Cross and Blue Shield
of Kansas
P.O. Box 239
1133 Topeka Ave.
Topeka, KS 66601

Kentucky
Blue Cross and Blue Shield
of Kentucky, Inc.
9901 Linn Station Rd.
Louisville, KY 40223

Louisiana
Blue Cross of Louisiana
P.O. Box 15699
10225 Florida Blvd.
Baton Rouge, LA 70895

Maine
Blue Cross and Blue Shield
of Maine
110 Free St.
Portland, ME 04101

Maryland
Blue Cross of Maryland,
Inc.
P.O. Box 9836
700 E. Joppa Rd.
Baltimore, MD 21204

Massachusetts
Blue Cross and Blue Shield
of Massachusetts, Inc.
100 Summer St.
Boston, MA 02106

Michigan
Blue Cross and Blue Shield
of Michigan
600 Lafayette E.
Detroit, MI 48226

Minnesota
Blue Cross and Blue Shield
of Minnesota
P.O. Box 43560
3535 Blue Cross Rd.
St. Paul, MN 55164

Mississippi
Blue Cross and Blue Shield
of Mississippi, Inc.
P.O. Box 1043
Lakeland Drive–East at
Flynt
Jackson, MS 39205

Missouri
Blue Cross Hospital
Service, Inc. of Missouri
4444 Forest Park Blvd.
St. Louis, MO 63108

Blue Cross of Kansas City
P.O. Box 169
3637 Broadway
Kansas City, MO 64141

St. Louis Blue Shield
(Missouri Medical
Service)
4444 Forest Park Blvd.
St. Louis, MO 63108

Montana
Blue Cross of Montana
P.O. Box 5004
3360 Tenth Ave., South
Great Falls, MT 59405

Blue Shield of Montana
(Montana Physician's
Service)
Box 4309
404 Fuller Ave.
Helena, MT 59601

Nebraska
Blue Cross and Blue Shield of Nebraska
P.O. Box 3248
Main P.O. Station
Omaha, NE 68180

Nevada
Blue Shield of Nevada
P.O. Box 10330
4600 Kietzke Ln.
Reno, NV 89502

New Hampshire
New Hampshire-Vermont Health Service
2 Pillsbury St.
Concord, NH 03301

New Jersey
Hospital Service Plan of New Jersey
P.O. Box 420
33 Washington St.
Newark, NJ 07102

Medical-Surgical Plan of New Jersey
33 Washington St.
Newark, NJ 07102

New Mexico
New Mexico Blue Cross and Blue Shield, Inc.
12800 Indian School Road, NE
Albuquerque, NM 87112

New York
Blue Cross of Central New York, Inc.
P.O. Box 4809
344 S. Warren St.
Syracuse, NY 13202

Blue Cross and Blue Shield of Greater New York
P.O. Box 345
Grand Central Station
New York, NY 10017

Blue Cross of Northeastern New York, Inc.
P.O. Box 8650
1251 New Scotland Rd.
Albany, NY 12208

Blue Cross of Western New York, Inc.
298 Main St.
Buffalo, NY 14202

Genesse Valley Medical Care, Inc.
41 Chestnut St.
Rochester, NY 14647

Hospital Plan, Inc.
5 Hopper St.
Utica, NY 13501

Hospital Service Corporation of Jefferson County
Box 570
158 Stone St.
Watertown, NY 13601

Medical and Surgical Care, Inc.
245 Genesee St.
Utica, NY 13501

Rochester Hospital Service Corporation
41 Chestnut St.
Rochester, NY 14647

North Carolina
Blue Cross and Blue Shield of North Carolina
P.O. Box 2291
5901 Chapel Hill–Durham Blvd.
Durham, NC 27702

North Dakota
Blue Cross of North Dakota
4510 Thirteenth Ave., SW
Fargo, ND 58121

Ohio
Blue Cross in Canton
Box 8590
4150 Belden Village St., NW
Canton, OH 44718

Blue Cross of Central Ohio
Box 16526
255 E. Main St.
Columbus, OH 43215

Blue Cross in Eastern Ohio
2400 Market St.
Youngstown, OH 44507

Blue Cross in Lima
Box 1046
50 Town Square
Lima, OH 45802

Blue Cross of Northeast Ohio
2066 E. Ninth St.
Cleveland, OH 44115

Blue Cross of Northwest Ohio
P.O. Box 943
3737 Sylvania Ave.
Toledo, OH 43656

Blue Cross in Southwest Ohio
1351 William Howard Taft Rd.
Cincinnati, OH 45206

Hospital Care Corporation
1351 William Howard Taft Rd.
Cincinnati, OH 45206

Medical Mutual of Cleveland, Inc.
2060 E. Ninth St.
Cleveland, OH 44115

Ohio Medical Indemnity Mutual Corp.
6740 N. Hight St.
Worthington, OH 43085

Oklahoma
Blue Cross and Blue Shield of Oklahoma (Group Hospital Service)
P.O. Box 3283
1215 S. Boulder Ave.
Tulsa, OK 74119

Oregon
Blue Cross of Oregon
P.O. Box 1271
100 SW Market St.
Portland, OR 97201

Pennsylvania
Blue Cross of Greater Philadelphia
1333 Chestnut St.
Philadelphia, PA 19107

Blue Cross of Lehigh Valley
1221 Hamilton St.
Allentown, PA 18102

Blue Cross of Northeastern Pennsylvania
70 N. Main St.
Wilkes-Barre, PA 18711

Blue Cross of Western Pennsylvania
1 Smithfield St.
Pittsburgh, PA 15222

Capital Blue Cross
100 Pine St.
Harrisburg, PA 17101

Pennsylvania Blue Shield
Camp Hill, PA 17011

Rhode Island
Blue Cross and Blue Shield of Rhode Island
444 Westminster Mall
Providence, RI 02901

South Carolina
Blue Cross and Blue Shield of South Carolina
I-20 East at Alpine Rd.
Columbia, SC 29219

South Dakota
See Iowa

Tennessee
Blue Cross and Blue Shield of Tennessee
801 Pine St.
Chattanooga, TN 37402

Memphis Hospital Service and Surgical Association, Inc.
P.O. Box 98
85 N. Danny Thomas Blvd.
Memphis, TN 38101

Texas
Group Hospital Service, Inc.
P.O. Box 225730
Main at North Central Expressway
Dallas, TX 75201

Utah
Blue Cross and Blue Shield of Utah
P.O. Box 30270
2455 Parley's Way
Salt Lake City, UT 84130

Vermont
See New Hampshire

Virginia
Blue Cross of Southwestern Virginia
P.O. Box 13047
3959 Electric Rd., SW
Roanoke, VA 24045

Blue Cross of Virginia
P.O. Box 27401
2015 Staples Mill Rd.
Richmond, VA 23230

Washington
Blue Cross of Washington and Alaska
P.O. Box 327
15700 Dayton Ave., North
Seattle, WA 98111

Chelan County Medical Service Corporation
Box 580
707 N. Emerson
Wenatchee, WA 98801

King County Medical Blue Shield
Box 21267
1800 Terry Ave.
Seattle, WA 98101

Medical Service Corporation for Eastern Washington
P.O. Box 3048
Terminal Annex
Spokane, WA 99202

Pierce County Medical Bureau, Inc.
1114 Broadway Plaza
Tacoma, WA 98402

Washington Physicians' Service
Fourth and Battery Bldg.
Suite 600
2401 Fourth Ave.
Seattle, WA 98121

West Virginia
Blue Cross Hospital Service, Inc.
P.O. Box 1353
Commerce Square
Charleston, WV 25325

Blue Cross of Northern West Virginia, Inc.
P.O. Box 7026
Twentieth and Chapline Streets
Wheeling, WV 26003

Blue Cross of West Central West Virginia
P.O. Box 1948
Seventh and Market Streets
Parkersburg, WV 26101

Morgantown Medical-Surgical Service, Inc.
265 High St.
Morgantown, WV 26505

Wisconsin
Blue Cross and Blue Shield of Wisconsin
P.O. Box 2025
401 W. Michigan St.
Milwaukee, WI 53201

Wyoming
Blue Cross and Blue Shield of Wyoming
P.O. Box 2266
400 House Ave.
Cheyenne, WY 82001

Alabama
Medical Services Administration
2500 Fairlane Dr.
Montgomery, AL 36130

Alaska
Division of Public Assistance
Department of Health and Social Services
Pouch H-07
Juneau, AK 99811

Arizona
Division of Medical Assistance
State Department Bldg.
1740 W. Adams St.
Phoenix, AZ 85001

Arkansas
Office of Medical Services
Arkansas Social Services
P.O. Box 1437
Little Rock, AR 72203

California
Medi-Cal Division
Department of Health Services
714P St.
Room 1253
Sacramento, CA 95814

Colorado
Division of Medical Assistance
Department of Social Services
1575 Sherman Ave.
Denver, CO 80203

Connecticut
Medical Care Administration
Department of Income Maintenance-Medicaid Program
110 Bartholomew Ave.
Hartford, CT 06106

Delaware
Medical Assistance Services
Department of Health and Social Services
Delaware State Hospital
New Castle, DE 19720

District of Columbia
District Medicaid Claims Processing
Department of Human Services
P.O. Box 37443
Washington, DC 20013

Florida
Medical Services
Department of Health and Rehabilitative Services
1323 Winewood Blvd.
Tallahassee, FL 32301

Georgia
Department of Medical Assistance
1010 W. Peachtree St., NW
Atlanta, GA 30309

Hawaii
Department of Social Service and Housing
P.O. Box 339
Honolulu, HI 96809

Idaho
Department of Health and Welfare
Statehouse
Boise, ID 83720

Illinois
Department of Public Aid
931 E. Washington St.
Springfield, IL 62762

Indiana
State Department of Public Welfare
100 N. Senate Ave.
Room 701
Indianapolis, IN 46204

Iowa
Medical Services Section
Department of Social
Services
Hoover State Office Bldg.
Fifth Floor
Des Moines, IA 50319

Kansas
Medical Services Section
Department of Social and
Rehabilitative Services
State Office Bldg.
Sixth Floor
Topeka, KS 66612

Kentucky
Division for Medical
Assistance
Bureau of Social Insurance
DHR Bldg.
Third Floor
275 E. Main St.
Frankfort, KY 40601

Louisiana
Medical Assistance
Program
Offices of Family Security
P.O. Box 44065
Baton Rouge, LA 70806

Maine
Bureau of Medical
Services
Department of Human
Services
Statehouse
Augusta, ME 04333

Maryland
Department of Health and
Mental Hygiene
201 W. Preston St.
Baltimore, MD 21201

Massachusetts
Department of Public
Welfare
600 Washington St.
Boston, MA 02111

Michigan
Medical Services
Administration
Department of Social
Services
921 W. Holmes
P.O. Box 30037
Lansing, MI 48909

Minnesota
Department of Public
Welfare
Centennial Office Bldg.
658 Cedar St.
St. Paul, MN 55155

Mississippi
Medicaid Commission
P.O. Box 16786
4785 I-55 North
Jackson, MS 39206

Missouri
Division of Family Services
Department of Social
Services
Broadway State Office Bldg.
P.O. Box 98
Jefferson City, MO 65101

Montana
Medical Assistance Bureau
Department of Social and
Rehabilitative Services
P.O. Box 4210
Helena, MT 59601

Nebraska
Department of Public
Welfare
301 Centennial Mall-South
Fifth Floor
Lincoln, NE 68509

Nevada
Medical Care Section
(Title XIX)
Welfare Division
251 Jeanell Dr.
Capitol Complex
Carson City, NV 89710

New Hampshire
Office of Medical Services
Department of Health and Welfare Services
Hazen Dr.
Concord, NH 03301

New Jersey
Division of Medical Assistance and Health Services
Department of Human Services
324 E. State St.
Trenton, NJ 08625

New Mexico
Medical Assistance Division
Department of Human Services
P.O. Box 2348
Santa Fe, NM 87503

New York
New York State Department of Social Services
Ten Eyck Office Bldg.
40 N. Pearl St.
Albany, NY 12243

North Carolina
Department of Human Resources
325 N. Salisbury St.
Raleigh, NC 27611

North Dakota
Social Service Board of North Dakota
State Capitol Bldg.
Bismarck, ND 58505

Ohio
Department of Public Welfare
Division of Medical Assistance
30 E. Broad St.
Thirty-second Floor
Columbus, OH 43215

Oklahoma
Department of Human Services
P.O. Box 25352
Oklahoma City, OK 73125

Oregon
Adult and Family Services Division
Department of Human Resources
203 Public Service Bldg.
Salem, OR 97310

Pennsylvania
Medical Assistance
Department of Public Welfare
Health and Welfare Bldg.
Room 515
Harrisburg, PA 17120

Rhode Island
Department of Social and Rehabilitative Services
600 New London Ave.
Cranston, RI 02920

South Carolina
Department of Social Services
P.O. Box 1520
Columbia, SC 29202

South Dakota
Office of Medical Services
Department of Social Services
Kneip Bldg.
Pierre, SD 57501

Tennessee
Bureau of Medicaid Administration
Department of Public Health
344 Cordell Hull Bldg.
Sixth Ave. North
Nashville, TN 37219

Texas
Department of Human Resources
P.O. Box 2960
Austin, TX 78769

Utah
Department of Health-
Division of Health Care
Financing and Standards
Medical Claims Unit
150 West North Temple
Salt Lake City, UT 84103

Vermont
Division of Medical
Services
Department of Social
Welfare
103 S. Main St.
Waterbury, VT 05676

Virginia
Medical Assistance Program
State Department of
Health
109 Governor St.
Richmond, VA 23219

Washington
Division of Medical
Assistance
Department of Social and
Health Services
Mail Stop LK-11
Olympia, WA 98504

West Virginia
Division of Medical Care
State Department of
Welfare
1900 Washington St., East
Charleston, WV 25305

Wisconsin
Bureau of Health Care
Financing
Department of Health and
Social Services
1 W. Wilson St.
Room 325
Madison, WI 53702

Wyoming
Department of Health and
Social Services
417 Hathaway Bldg.
Cheyenne, WY 82002

Appendix 18. Drug Enforcement Administration: Regional, District, and Resident Offices

Northeast

Northeastern Regional Office
555 W. Fifty-seventh St.
New York, NY 10019
212-399-5131

Boston District Office
JFK Federal Bldg.
Room G-64
Boston, MA 02203
617-223-2170

Buffalo Resident Office
268 Main St.
Suite 300
Buffalo, NY 14202
716-846-4421

Hartford District Office
450 Main St.
Room 628-E
Hartford, CT 06102
203-244-3230

Long Island District Office
1 Huntington Quadrangle
Suite 1C-02
Melville, NY 11746
516-420-4500

Newark District Office
Federal Office Bldg.
970 Broad St.
Newark, NJ 07101
201-645-6060

New York City District Office
555 W. Fifty-seventh St.
New York, NY 10019
212-399-5018

Philadelphia District Office
William J. Green Federal Bldg.
600 Arch St.
Room 10224
Philadelphia, PA 19106
215-597-9540

Pittsburgh District Office
Federal Building
1000 Liberty Ave.
Room 2306
Pittsburgh, PA 15222
412-644-3390

Southeast

Southeastern Regional Office
8400 NW Fifty-third St.
Miami, FL 33166
305-591-4880

Atlanta District Office
United Family Life Building
230 Houston St., NE
Suite 200
Atlanta, GA 30303
404-221-4412

Baltimore District Office
955 Federal Bldg.
31 Hopkins Plaza
Baltimore, MD 21202
301-962-2224

Birmingham Resident Office
236 Goodwin Crest
Suite 520
Birmingham, AL 35209
205-229-0620

Greensboro Resident Office
925 W. Market St.
Room 111
Greensboro, NC 27401
919-378-5208

Miami District Office
8400 NW Fifty-third St.
Miami, FL 33166
305-591-4980

Nashville Resident Office
Estes KeFauver Federal Bldg.
Room A929
801 Broadway
Nashville, TN 37202
615-251-5988

New Orleans District Office
1001 Howard Ave.
New Orleans, LA 70113
504-589-2171

Tampa Resident Office
700 Twiggs St.
Suite 400
Tampa, FL 33602
813-228-2178

North Central

North Central Regional Office
1800 Dirksen Federal Bldg.
219 S. Dearborn St.
Chicago, IL 60604
312-353-1234

Chicago District Office
1800 Dirksen Federal Bldg.
219 S. Dearborn St.
Chicago, IL 60604
312-353-1234

Cincinnati District Office
Federal Office Bldg.
550 Main St.
Room 7405
Cincinnati, OH 45202
518-684-3571

Cleveland District Office
601 Rockwell
Room 300
Cleveland, OH 44114
216-293-3705

Des Moines Resident Office
U.S. Courthouse
P.O. Box 1784
Des Moines, IA 50309
515-862-4700

Detroit District Office
357 Federal Bldg.
231 W. Lafayette
Detroit, MI 48226
313-226-7290

Indianapolis Resident Office
575 N. Pennsylvania
Room 290
Indianapolis, IN 46204
317-331-7977

Kansas City District Office
U.S. Courthouse
1150 Grand Ave.
Suite 400
Kansas City, MO 64106
816-758-2621

Minneapolis Resident Office
Federal Bldg.
110 S. Fourth St.
Room 402
Minneapolis, MN 55401
612-725-2783

St. Louis District Office
Chromaloy Plaza
Suite 200
120 S. Central Ave.
St. Louis, MO 63105
314-279-3264

South Central

South Central Regional Office
1880 Regal Row
Dallas, TX 75235
214-767-7203

Dallas District Office
1880 Regal Row
Dallas TX 75235
214-767-7203

Denver District Office
U.S. Custom House
Room 316
P.O. Box 1860
Denver, CO 80201
303-837-3951

Phoenix District Office
Valley Bank Center
201 N. Central
Suite 1980
Phoenix, AZ 85073
602-261-4866

West

Western Regional Office
350 S. Figueroa St.
Suite 800
Los Angeles, CA 90071
213-688-5225

Honolulu Resident Office
FAA Bldg.
Fourth Floor
1833 Kalakaua Ave.
Honolulu, HI 96815
808-556-9000 (Ask for 556-8391

Los Angeles District Office
350 S. Figueroa St.
Suite 800
Los Angeles, CA 90071
213-688-5225

Portland Resident Office
Terminal Sales Bldg.
1220 SW Morrison
Suite 706
Portland, OR 97205
503-423-3371

San Francisco District Office
450 Golden Gate Ave.
Box 36035
San Francisco, CA 94102
415-556-3325

Seattle District Office
221 First Ave. West
Suite 200
Seattle, WA 98119
206-399-5996

Dictaphone Corp.
120 Old Post Rd.
Rye, NY 10580
914-967-6211

IBM Corp.
Parson's Pond Dr.
Franklin Lakes, NJ 07417
201-848-1900

Lanier Business Products
1700 Chantilly Dr., NE
Atlanta, GA 30324
404-329-8000

Norelco Corp.
Phillips Business Systems, Inc.
810 Woodbury Rd.
Woodbury, NY 11797
516-921-9310

Sanyo Business Systems Corp.
51 Joseph St.
Moonachie, NJ 07074
201-440-9300

Sony Corp. of America
9 W. Fifty-seventh St.
New York, NY 10019
212-371-5800

Business Systems &
Security Marketing
Association, Inc.
835 S. 130th St.
Omaha, NE 68154
402-333-6780

Hon, Inc.
414 E. Third St.
Muschatine, IA 52761
319-264-7100

Kardex Systems, Inc.
P.O. Box 171
Marietta, Ohio 45750
800-848-9761

Lundia Myers Industries,
Inc.
600 Capitol Way
Jacksonville, IL 62650
217-243-8585

Steelcase Corp.
1120 Thirty-sixth St.
Grand Rapids, MI 49508
616-274-2710

Supreme Equipment &
Systems Corp.
170 Fifty-third St.
Brooklyn, NY 11232
212-492-7777

Tab Products Corp.
269 Hanover
Palo Alto, CA 94300
415-493-5790

White Power Files, Inc.
850 Springfield Rd.
Union, NJ 07083
201-687-9522

Region 1 (Connecticut, Maine, Massachusetts, New Hampshire, Rhode Island, and Vermont)

Department of Labor
1630 JFK Federal Bldg.
Government Center
Boston, MA 02203
617-223-6761

Region 2 (New Jersey and New York)

Department of Labor
Suite 3400
1515 Broadway
1 Astor Plaza
New York, NY 10036
212-971-5405

Region 3 (Delaware, District of Columbia, Maryland, Pennsylvania, Virginia, and West Virginia)

Department of Labor
3535 Market St.
P.O. Box 13309
Philadelphia, PA 19104
215-595-1154

Region 4 (Alabama, Florida, Georgia, Kentucky, Mississippi, North Carolina, South Carolina, and Tennessee)

Department of Labor
Suite 540
1371 Peachtree St., NE
Atlanta, GA 30309
404-881-4951

Region 5 (Illinois, Indiana, Minnesota, Michigan, Ohio, and Wisconsin)

Department of Labor
230 S. Dearborn St.
Ninth Floor
Chicago, IL 60604
312-353-1880

Region 6 (Arkansas, Louisiana, New Mexico, Oklahoma, and Texas)

Department of Labor
555 Griffin Square Bldg.
Second Floor
Dallas, TX 75202
214-749-3516

Region 7 (Iowa, Kansas, Missouri, and Nebraska)

Department of Labor
911 Walnut St.
Fifteenth Floor
Kansas City, MO 64106
816-374-2481

Region 8 (Colorado, Montana, North Dakota, South Dakota, Utah, and Wyoming)

Department of Labor
Federal Bldg.
1961 Stout St.
Denver, CO 80294
303-837-5516

Region 9 (Arizona, California, Hawaii, and Nevada)

Department of Labor
450 Golden Gate Ave.
Box 36017
San Francisco, CA 94102
415-556-4678

Region 10 (Alaska, Idaho, Oregon, and Washington)

Department of Labor
300 W. Harrison St.
Seattle, WA 98174
206-464-7870

Alabama
Department of Industrial Relations
Industrial Relations Bldg.
Montgomery, AL 36130
205-832-5040

Alaska
Department of Labor
P.O. Box 1149
Juneau, AK 99811
907-465-2700

Arizona
Industrial Commission
1610 W. Jefferson
P.O. Box 19070
Phoenix, AZ 85005
602-255-4661

Arkansas
Workers' Compensation Commission
Justice Bldg.
State Capitol Grounds
Little Rock, AR 72201
501-372-3930

California
Division of Industrial Accidents
525 Golden Gate Ave.
San Francisco, CA 94101
415-557-0391

Colorado
Department of Labor and Employment
251 E. Twelfth Ave.
Denver, CO 80203
303-866-6213

Connecticut
Workers' Compensation Commission
295 Treadwell St.
Hamden, CT 06514
203-789-7783

Delaware
Industrial Accident Board
State Office Bldg.
Sixth Floor
820 N. French St.
Wilmington, DE 19801
302-571-2884

District of Columbia
District of Columbia Department of Employment Services
950 Upshur St., NW
Washington, DC 20011
202-724-3932

Florida
Division of Workers' Compensation
1321 Executive Center Dr., East
Tallahassee, FL 32301
904-488-6093

Georgia
Board of Workers' Compensation
1800 Peachtree St., NW
Atlanta, GA 30367
404-894-3082

Hawaii
Disability Compensation Division
Department of Labor and Industrial Relations
825 Mililani St.
Honolulu, HI 96813
808-548-2211

Idaho
Industrial Commission
317 Main St.
Boise, ID 83720
208-334-3250

Illinois
Industrial Commission
160 N. LaSalle St.
Chicago, IL 60601
312-793-2480

Indiana
Industrial Board
601 State Office Bldg.
100 N. Senate Ave.
Indianapolis, IN 46204
317-232-3808

Iowa
Industrial Commissioner
507 Tenth St.
Des Moines, IA 50307
515-281-5394

Kansas
Division of Workers' Compensation
535 Kansas Ave.
Sixth Floor
Topeka, KS 66603
913-296-3441

Kentucky
Workers' Compensation Board
127 S. Bldg.
Frankfort, KY 40601
502-564-5550

Louisiana
Department of Labor
1045 State Land and Natural Resources Bldg.
P.O. Box 44094
Baton Rouge, LA 70804
504-342-3111

Maine
Workers' Compensation Commission
State Office Bldg.
Augusta, ME 04333
207-289-3751

Maryland
Workers' Compensation Commission
108 E. Lexington St.
Baltimore, MD 21202
301-659-4700

Massachusetts
Industrial Accident Board
Leverett Saltonstall Office Bldg.
100 Cambridge St.
Boston, MA 02202
617-727-3407

Michigan
Bureau of Workers' Disability Compensation
Department of Labor
P.O. Box 30016
Lansing, MI 48909
517-373-3490

Minnesota
Department of Labor and Industry
444 Lafayette Road
St. Paul, MN 55101
612-296-6107

Mississippi
Workmens' Compensation Commission
1404 Walter Sillers State Office Bldg.
P.O. Box 987
Jackson, MS 39205
601-354-7496

Missouri
Division of Workers' Compensation
Department of Labor and Industrial Relations
P.O. Box 58
Jefferson City, MO 65102
314-751-4231

Montana
Division of Workers' Compensation
815 Front St.
Helena, MT 59601
406-449-2047

Nebraska
Workmen's Compensation Court
State Capitol
Lincoln, NE 68509
402-471-2568

Nevada
Industrial Commission
515 E. Musser Street
Carson City, NV 89714
702-885-5220

New Hampshire
Department of Labor
19 Pillsbury St.
Concord, NH 03301
603-271-3176

New Jersey
Department of Labor and Industry
John Fitch Plaza
Trenton, NJ 08625
609-292-2121

New Mexico
Labor and Industrial Commission
509 Camino de Los Marquez
Santa Fe, NM 87501
505-827-2756

New York
Workers' Compensation Board
2 World Trade Center
New York, NY 10047
212-944-3356

North Carolina
Industrial Commission
Dobbs Bldg.
430 N. Salisbury St.
Raleigh, NC 27611
919-733-4820

North Dakota
Workmen's Compensation Bureau
Russell Bldg.
Highway 83 North
Bismarck, ND 58505
701-224-2700

Ohio
Industrial Commission of Ohio
246 N. High St.
Columbus, OH 43215
614-466-6136

Oklahoma
Workers' Compensation Court
Jim Thorpe Bldg.
P.O. Box 53038
Oklahoma City, OK 73105
405-521-8025

Oregon
Workers' Compensation Department
Labor and Industries Bldg.
Salem, OR 97310
503-378-3302

Pennsylvania
Bureau of Workers' Compensation
3607 Derry St.
Harrisburg, PA 17111
717-783-5421

Rhode Island
Workers' Compensation Commission
25 Canal St.
Providence, RI 02903
401-277-3097

South Carolina
Industrial Commission
Middleburg Office Park
1800 St. Julian Pl.
Columbia, SC 29204
803-758-2556

South Dakota
Department of Labor
Division of Labor and Management
Joe Foss Bldg.
Room 425
Pierre, SD 57501
605-773-3681

Tennessee
Division of Workers' Compensation
Department of Labor
501 Union Bldg.
Second Floor
Nashville, TN 37219
615-741-2395

Texas
Industrial Accident Board
200 E. Riverside Dr.
Austin, TX 78704
512-475-2251

Utah
Industrial Commission
350 E. 500 South
Salt Lake City, UT 84111
801-533-5971

Vermont
Department of Labor and Industry
Montpelier, VT 05602
802-828-2286

Virginia
Industrial Commission
Blanton Bldg.
Richmond, VA 23214
804-786-3651

Washington
Department of Labor and Industries
General Administration Bldg.
Olympia, WA 98504
206-753-6341

West Virginia
Workmen's Compensation Fund
112 California Ave.
Charleston, WV 25305
304-348-2580

Wisconsin
Department of Industry, Labor, and Human Relations
201 E. Washington Ave.
P.O. Box 7398
Madison, WI 53709
608-266-7552

Wyoming
Workers' Compensation Division
2305 Carey Ave.
Cheyenne, WY 82002
307-777-7441

1. Blue Cross/Blue Shield of South Carolina, I-20 at Alpine, Columbia, SC 29219, is the CHAMPUS fiscal intermediary for the following states:

Delaware	South Carolina
District of Columbia	Virginia
Maryland	North Carolina
Pennsylvania	

2. Blue Shield of California, CHAMPUS/CHAMPVA Program, P.O. Box 85024, San Diego, CA 92138, is the CHAMPUS fiscal intermediary for the following states:

Arizona	Michigan
California	Nevada
Connecticut	New Hampshire
Florida	New Mexico
Maine	Puerto Rico
Massachusetts	Vermont

3. Hawaii Medical Service Association, P.O. Box 860, Honolulu, HI 96808, is the CHAMPUS fiscal intermediary for Hawaii.

4. Mutual of Omaha Insurance Company, CHAMPUS/CHAMPVA Program, Mutual of Omaha Plaza, Omaha, NB 68175, is the CHAMPUS fiscal intermediary for the following states:

Alabama	Nebraska
Colorado	Ohio
Georgia	West Virginia
Mississippi	

5. Blue Cross of Rhode Island, CHAMPUS/CHAMPVA Program, 1 Weybosset Hill, Providence, RI 02903, is the CHAMPUS fiscal intermediary for the following states:

New Jersey	Rhode Island
New York	

6. Blue Cross/Blue Shield of Tennessee, CHAMPUS/CHAMPVA Program, 730 Chestnut Street, Chattanooga, TN 37402, is the CHAMPUS fiscal intermediary for Tennessee.

7. Blue Cross of Washington-Alaska, P.O. Box 77084, Seattle, WA 98177, is the CHAMPUS fiscal intermediary for the following states:

Alaska	Utah
Idaho	Washington
Montana	Wyoming
Oregon	

8. Wisconsin Physicians' Service, P.O. Box 7927, Madison, WI 53707, is the CHAMPUS fiscal intermediary for the following states:

   Arkansas
   Illinois
   Indiana
   Iowa
   Kansas
   Kentucky
   Louisiana
   Minnesota
   Missouri
   North Dakota
   Oklahoma
   South Dakota
   Texas
   Wisconsin

Bibbero Systems, Inc.
109 Stevenson
Third Floor
San Francisco, CA 94105

Black & Skaggs Associates
Box 1130
1201 Security National Bank Bldg.
Battle Creek, MI 49016

Business Envelope Manufacturers, Inc.
900 Grand Blvd.
Deep Park, NY 11729

The Colwell Company
201 Kenyon Rd.
Champaign, IL 61820

Control-o-Fax/Creative Systems, Inc.
Box 778
3070 W. Airline Highway
Waterloo, IA 50704

The Drawing Board, Inc.
Box 220505
256 Regal Rd.
Dallas, TX 75222

Histacount Corp.
Walt Whitman Rd.
Melville, NY 11747

McBee Systems
600 Washington Ave.
Carlstadt, NJ 07072

Medical Arts Press
3440 Winnetka Ave., North
Minneapolis, MN 55427

Milcom
Miller Communications, Inc.
322 Westport Ave.
Norwalk, CT 06856

Orion Systems
422 Oakmead Pkwy.
Sunneyvale, CA 94086

Physicians' Record Co.
3000 S. Ridgeland Ave.
Berwyn, IL 60402

Safeguard Business Systems
400 Maryland Dr.
Fort Washington, PA 19034

The Shingles System
422 Oakmead Pkwy.
Sunnyvale, CA 94086

Appendix 25. Small Claims Courts

State	Common Name	Maximum Claim
Alabama	Small Claims Division of District Court	$ 500
Alaska	Small Claims Court of the District Court	2,000
Arizona	Justice of Peace Court	1,000
Arkansas	Small Claims Division of Municipal or Justice Court	300
California	Small Claims Division of Municipal or Justice Court	750
Colorado	Small Claims Division of County Court	500
Connecticut	Small Claims Division of Superior Court	750
Delaware	Justice of Peace Court	1,500
District of Columbia	Small Claims Branch of D.C. Superior Court	750
Florida	Summary Claims Division of County Court	1,500
Georgia[1]	—	—
Hawaii	Small Claims Division of District Court	1,000
Idaho	Small Claims Department of District Court	1,000
Illinois[2]	Small Claims Court, or *Pro Se Court* (Cook County)	—
Indiana	Small Claims Court	3,000
Iowa	Small Claims Division of District Court	1,000
Kansas	Small Claims Court	500
Kentucky	Small Claims Division of District Court	1,000
Louisiana	Small Claims Division of City Court or Justice of Peace Court	750
Maine	Small Claims Division of District Court	800
Maryland	Small Claims Division of District Court	500
Massachusetts	Small Claims Division of District Court or Municipal Court	750
Michigan[3]	Small Claims Division of District Court	600
Minnesota	Conciliation Court	1,000
Mississippi	Justice of Peace Court	500
Missouri	Small Claims Court of Circuit Court	500
Montana	Small Claims Division of Justice of Peace Court	750
Nebraska	Small Claims Division of Municipal or County Court	1,000
Nevada	Justice Court	750
New Hampshire	Small Claims Court of Municipal or District Court	500
New Jersey	Small Claims Court of County District Court	500
New Mexico	Small Claims Court	2,000
New York	Small Claims Court	1,000
North Carolina	Small Claims Court of Magistrate's Court	800
North Dakota[4]	Small Claims Court of Justice or County Court	—
Ohio	Small Claims Court	500

Appendix 25 (Continued)

State	*Common Name*	*Maximum Claim*
Oklahoma	Small Claims Division of District Court	$ 600
Oregon	Small Claims Division of District Court	700
Pennsylvania	District Justice Court or Municipal Court (Philadelphia only)	2,000
Rhode Island	Small Claims Division of District Court	500
South Carolina	Magistrate's Court	1,000
South Dakota	Small Claims Division of Magistrate's Court	2,000
Tennessee	General Sessions Court	5,000
Texas	Small Claims Court of Justice of Peace Court	500
Utah	Small Claims Court of Circuit or Justice Court	400
Vermont	Small Claims Division of District Court	500
Virginia[5]	General District Court	1,000
Washington	Small Claims Court	500
West Virginia	Magistrate's Court	1,500
Wisconsin	Small Claims Court of Circuit Court	1,000
Wyoming	Justice of Peace Court	750

[1] Georgia does not have a statewide system of small claims courts; many counties have small claims courts with varying claim limits, fees, and procedures.
[2] Illinois fees and procedures vary from circuit to circuit. The general small claims limit throughout the state is $1,000, but in Cook County there is a special court called *Pro Se* Court of Circuit Court in which the claim limit is $500.
[3] Michigan has 28 cities with municipal small claims courts rather than district courts. In the municipal courts, the maximum claim is $1,500 and the court procedures are more complex.
[4] Some North Dakota counties have County Justice Courts in which the maximum claim is $500. Seventeen other counties have County Courts of Increased Jurisdiction in which the maximum claim is $1,000.
[5] In Virginia, if the amount involved is greater than $1,000 and the defendant files an affidavit with the court indicating a substantial defense, and pays accrued court costs, the case will be transferred to the Circuit Court.

Alabama	800-292-6300
Alaska	See local directory
Arizona	800-352-6911
Arkansas	800-482-9350
California	Call the telephone number shown in the white pages of your local telephone directory under U.S. Government, Internal Revenue Service, Federal Tax Assistance
Colorado	800-332-2060
Connecticut	800-842-1120
Delaware	800-292-9575
District of Columbia	202-488-3100
Florida	800-342-8300
Georgia	800-222-1040
Hawaii	808-935-4895
Idaho	800-632-5990
Illinois	800-252-2921
Indiana	800-382-9740
Iowa	800-362-2600
Kansas	800-362-2190
Kentucky	800-292-6570
Louisiana	800-362-6900
Maine	800-452-8750
Maryland	800-492-0460
Massachusetts	800-392-6288
Michigan	800-482-0670
Minnesota	800-652-9062
Mississippi	800-241-3868
Missouri	800-392-4200
Montana	800-332-2275
Nebraska	800-642-9960
Nevada	800-492-6552
New Hampshire	800-582-7200
New Jersey	800-242-6750
New Mexico	800-527-3880
New York	800-342-3799 or 800-462-1560
North Carolina	800-822-8800
North Dakota	800-342-4710
Ohio	800-362-9050
Oklahoma	800-962-3456
Oregon	800-452-1980
Pennsylvania	800-242-0250
Rhode Island	See local directory
South Carolina	800-241-3868
South Dakota	800-592-1870

Tennessee	800-342-8420
Texas	800-492-4830
Utah	800-662-5370
Vermont	800-642-3110
Virginia	800-552-9500
Washington	800-732-1040
West Virginia	800-642-1931
Wisconsin	800-452-9100
Wyoming	800-525-6060

If your principal office is located in	File your application for an Employee Identification number at
New Jersey, New York City, counties of Nassau, Rockland, Suffolk, or Westchester	Holtsville, NY 00501
New York (all other counties), Connecticut, Maine, Massachusetts, New Hampshire, Rhode Island, or Vermont	Andover, MA 05501
Delaware, District of Columbia, Maryland, or Pennsylvania	Philadelphia, PA 19255
Alabama, Florida, Georgia, Mississippi, or South Carolina	Atlanta, GA 31101
Michigan or Ohio	Cincinnati, OH 45999
Arkansas, Kansas, Louisiana, New Mexico, Oklahoma, or Texas	Austin, TX 73301
Alaska, Arizona, Colorado, Idaho, Minnesota, Montana, Nebraska, Nevada, North Dakota, Oregon, South Dakota, Utah, Washington, or Wyoming	Ogden, UT 84201
Illinois, Iowa, Missouri, or Wisconsin	Kansas City, MO 64999
California or Hawaii	Fresno, CA 93888
Indiana, Kentucky, North Carolina, Tennessee, Virginia, or West Virginia	Memphis, TN 37501

Note: File on IRS Form SS-4 with the Internal Revenue Service Center.

State	Court of Jurisdiction	Time Limit for Filing Claims (months)	Dated from[1]
Alabama	Probate Court	6	A
Alaska	Probate Court	6	B
Arizona	Probate Court	4	B
Arkansas	Probate Court	6	B
California	Superior Court	4	A
Colorado[2]	District Court	6	B
Connecticut	Probate Court	variable	F
Delaware	Court of Chancery	6	B
District of Columbia	Probate Court	3	B
Florida	Probate Court	3	B
Georgia	Probate Court	3	B
Hawaii	Circuit Court	4	B
Idaho	District Court (Magistrate Division)	4	B
Illinois	Circuit Court	6	A
Indiana	Circuit Court	5	B
Iowa	District Court	6	C
Kansas	District Court	6	B
Kentucky	District Court	6	A
Louisiana	District Court	3	E
Maine	Probate Court	4	A
Maryland	Orphan's Court	6	A
Massachusetts	Probate Court	4	A
Michigan	Probate Court	2	B
Minnesota[3]	Probate Court	4	B
Mississippi	Chancery Court	3	B
Missouri	Circuit Court Probate Division	6	B
Montana	District Court	4	B
Nebraska	County Court	2	B
Nevada[4]	District Court	—	B
New Hampshire	Probate Court	6	A
New Jersey[5]	Superior Court Chancery or Probate Division	6	—
New Mexico	District Court	2	B
New York	Surrogate Court	3	B
North Carolina	Superior Court	6	B
North Dakota	County Court	3	B
Ohio	Probate Court	4	B
Oklahoma	District Court	2	B

Appendix 28 (Continued)

State	Court of Jurisdiction	Time Limit for Filing Claims (months)	Dated from[1]
Oregon[6]	Circuit Court	4	B
Pennsylvania	Orphan's Court	12	E
Rhode Island	Probate Court	6	B
South Carolina	Probate Court	5	B
South Dakota	Circuit Court	2	B
Tennessee	Probate Court	6	B
Texas	Probate Court	6	A
Utah	District Court	3	B
Vermont	Probate Court	4	B
Virginia	Circuit Court	6	A
Washington	Superior Court	4	B
West Virginia	County Commissioner of Assets	variable	E
Wisconsin	County Court	3	A
Wyoming	District Court	3	B

Note: Attempts have been made to insure the accuracy of the information in this Appendix. The Attorney General's office of each state has been consulted, and the individual state statutes dealing with matters of probate have been researched. The author, however, disclaims responsibility for clerical errors, typographical errors, or legislative changes of state statutes dealing with courts of jurisdiction or time limits for filing claims. Your attorney should be consulted when filing claims against a deceased's estate.

[1] *A* = the date of issuance of letters of administration; *B* = the date of first public notice to creditors; *C* = the date of second public notice to creditors; *D* = the date of last public notice to creditors; *E* = the date of death; and *F* = the date set by the court.

[2] Colorado. In Denver and Colorado Springs the court of jurisdiction for matters of probate is the Probate Court. The court of jurisdiction in all other areas is the District Court.

[3] Minnesota. In Hennepin and Ramsey counties the court of jurisdiction for matters of probate is the County Court. The court of jurisdiction in all other counties is the Probate Court.

[4] Nevada. The time limit for filing claims against the estate of the deceased is two months if the estate is worth less than $60,000. The time limit for filing claims against the estate is ninety days if the estate is worth more than $60,000.

Adler-Royal Business
Machines, Inc.
150 New Park Ave.
Hartford, CT 06106
203-236-2354

Canon, Inc.
10 Nevada Dr.
Lake Success, NY 11042
516-468-6700

Eastman Kodak Co.
343 State St.
Rochester, NY 14608
716-325-2000

International Business
Machines Corp. (IBM)
590 Madison Ave.
New York, NY 10022
212-223-2500

Minolta Corp.
101 Williams Dr.
Ramsey, NY 07446
201-825-4000

Minnesota Mining &
Manufacturing Co. (3 M)
3 M Center
St. Paul, MN 55101
612-733-1110

Pitney Bowes, Inc.
Walter H. Wheeler, Jr., Dr.
Stamford, CT 06904
203-356-5000

Savin Corp.
Columbus Ave.
Valhalla, NY 10595
914-769-9500

Sharp Electronics Corp.
10 Keystone Pl.
Paramus, NJ 07642
201-265-5600

Xerox Corp.
800 Long Ridge Rd.
Stamford, CT 06904
203-329-8700

[5] New Jersey. The time limit for presenting claims against the estate of the deceased is measured from the date of entry of the court's order to present claims [N.J. Stat. Ann. Title 3A:24-3].

[6] Oregon. The court of jurisdiction for matters of probate is the County Court in Gilliam, Grant, Harney, Malheur, Sherman, and Wheeler counties.

Appendix 30. Federal Reserve Branch Banks

Atlanta
104 Marietta St., NW
Atlanta, GA 30303

Boston
30 Pearl St.
Boston, MA 02106

Chicago
230 S. LaSalle St.
Chicago, IL 60690

Cleveland
1455 E. Sixth St.
Cleveland, OH 44101

Dallas
400 S. Akard St.
Dallas, TX 75222

Kansas City
925 Grand Ave.
Kansas City, MO 63166

Minneapolis
250 Marquette Ave.
Minneapolis, MN 55480

New York
33 Liberty St.
New York, NY 10045

Philadelphia
925 Chestnut St.
Philadelphia, PA 19105

Richmond
100 N. Ninth St.
Richmond VA 23261

St. Louis
411 Locus St.
St. Louis, MO 63166

San Francisco
400 Sansome St.
San Francisco, CA 94120

Appendix 31. Brokerage Firms Offering Cash Management Services

Advest, Inc.
6 Central Row
Hartford, CT 06103
203-525-1421

Bache Group, Inc.
100 Gold St.
New York, NY 10038
212-791-1000

Dean, Witter, Reynolds, Inc.
130 Liberty St.
New York, NY 10006
212-437-3000

A. G. Edwards and Sons, Inc.
1 N. Jefferson St.
St. Louis, MO 63103
314-289-3000

Fidelity Corp.
82 Devonshire St.
Boston, MA 02109
800-225-8740

E. F. Hutton & Co. Inc.
1 Battery Park Plaza
New York, NY 10004
212-742-5000

Edward D. Jones & Co.
201 Progress Parkway
Hazelwood, MO 63043
314-576-0100

Charles Schwab & Co., Inc.
1 Second St.
San Francisco, CA 94105
415-546-1000

Shearson Loeb Rhodes, Inc.
14 Wall St.
New York, NY 10005
212-577-7000

Appendix 32. Institutions Offering Money Market Funds

Cash Reserve Management Fund
E. F. Hutton & Co., Inc.
1 Battery Park Plaza
New York, NY 10004
212-742-5000

Daily Cash Accumulation Fund
P.O. Box 300
Denver, CO 80201
800-525-9310

Dreyfus Liquid Assets Fund
767 Fifth Ave.
New York, NY 10022
800-223-5525

Fidelity Daily Income Fund
82 Devonshire St.
Boston, MA 02109
800-225-8740

InterCapital Liquid Assets Fund
Dean, Witter, Reynolds, Inc.
130 Liberty St.
New York, NY 10006
212-437-3000

Merrill Lynch Ready Asset Fund
Merrill Lynch & Co., Inc.
165 Broadway
New York, NY 10080
212-766-1212

Moneymart Assets Fund
Bache Group, Inc.
100 Gold St.
New York, NY 10038
212-791-1000

Reserve Fund
810 Seventh Ave.
New York, NY 10019
800-223-5547

Shearson Daily Dividend Fund
Shearson Loeb Rhodes, Inc.
14 Wall St.
New York, NY 10005
212-577-7000

Appendix 33. Manufacturers of Patient Education Materials

The following companies have patient education materials available including charts, skeletons, models, slides, transparencies, and preserved materials.

Armstrong Industries
3660 Commercial Ave.
P.O. Box 7
Northbrook, IL 60062

Clay Adams, Inc.
Webro Rd.
Parsippany, NJ 07054

Denoyer-Geppert Co.
5235 Ravenswood Ave.
Chicago, IL 60640

General Biological Supply House, Inc.
Division of MacMillan Science Co., Inc.
8200 S. Hoyne Ave.
Chicago, IL 60640

Medical Plastics Laboratory
P.O. Box 38
Gatersville, TX 76528

NASCO
901 Jonesville Ave.
Fort Atkinson, WI 53538

A. J. Nystrom Biological Model Co.
3333 N. Elstron Ave.
Chicago, IL 60618

Ward's Natural Science Establishment, Inc.
P.O. Box 1712
Rochester, NY 14603
or
P.O. Box 1749
Monterey, CA 93940

Atlanta
Federal Bldg.
Room 100
275 Peachtree St., NE
Atlanta, GA 30303
404-221-6947

Birmingham
9220 Parkway East-B
Roebuck Shopping City
Birmingham, AL 35206
205-254-1056

Boston
John F. Kennedy Federal Bldg.
Room G25
Sudbury St.
Boston, MA 02203
617-223-6071

Chicago
Everett McKinley Dirksen Bldg.
Room 1463
219 S. Dearborn St.
Chicago, IL 60604
312-353-5133

Cleveland
Federal Office Bldg.
First Floor
1240 E. Ninth St.
Cleveland, OH 44199
216-522-4922

Columbus
Federal Bldg.
Room 207
200 N. High St.
Columbus, OH 43215
614-469-6956

Dallas
Federal Bldg.
Room 1C50
1100 Commerce St.
Dallas, TX 75242
214-767-0076

Denver
Federal Bldg.
Room 117
1961 Stout St.
Denver, CO 80294
303-837-3964

Detroit
Patrick V. McNamara Federal Bldg.
Suite 160
477 Michigan Ave.
Detroit, MI 48226
313-226-7816

Houston
45 College Center
9319 Gulf Freeway
Houston, TX 77018
713-226-5453

Jacksonville
Federal Bldg.
Room 158
400 W. Bay St.
Jacksonville, FL 32202
904-791-3801

Kansas City
Federal Office Bldg.
Room 144
601 E. Twelfth St.
Kansas City, MO 64106
816-374-2160

Los Angeles
Federal Office Bldg.
Room 2039
300 N. Los Angeles St.
Los Angeles, CA 90012
213-688-5841

Milwaukee
Federal Bldg.
Room 190
519 E. Wisconsin Ave.
Milwaukee, WI 53202
414-291-1304

New York
26 Federal Plaza
Room 100
New York, NY 10007
212-264-3825

Philadelphia
Federal Office Bldg.
Room 1214
600 Arch St.
Philadelphia, PA 19106
215-597-0677

Pittsburgh
Federal Bldg.
Room 118
1000 Liberty Ave.
Pittsburgh, PA 15222
412-644-2721

Pueblo
Majestic Bldg.
720 N. Main St.
Pueblo, CO 81003
303-544-3142

San Francisco
Federal Office Bldg.
Room 1023
450 Golden Gate Ave.
San Francisco, CA 94102
415-556-0643

Seattle
Federal Office Bldg.
Room 194
915 Second Ave.
Seattle, WA 98174
206-399-4270

Washington, DC and Vicinity
Government Printing Office
710 N. Capitol St.
Washington, DC 20402
202-275-2091

Department of Commerce
Fourteenth & E Streets, NW
Room 1604
Washington, DC 20230
202-377-3527

Department of Health and Human Resources
330 Independence Ave., SW
Room 1528
Washington, DC 20201
202-472-7478

Department of State
Twenty-first and C Streets, NW
North Lobby
Room 2817
Washington, DC 20520
202-632-1437

International Communications Agency
1776 Pennsylvania Ave., NW
Washington, DC 20547
202-724-9928

Laurel Bookstore
8660 Cherry Ln.
Laurel, MD 20810
301-953-7974

Pentagon
Main Concourse, South End
Washington, DC 20310
703-557-1821

Appendix 35. Review Courses and Correspondence Services for FLEX and ECFMG Candidates

Review Courses

Program for foreign medical graduates
Office of the Internal Medical Education
University of Miami-School of Medicine
Miami, FL 33131

Comprehensive medical review courses
St. Barnabus Medical Center
Department of Medical Education
94 Old Short Hills Rd.
Livingston, NJ 07039

Medical review program
Center of Health Sciences
Oakland University
Rochester, MN 48063

FLEX review and ECFMG refresher course
Hahnemann Medical College and Hospital
School of Continuing Education
230 N. Broad St.
Philadelphia, PA 19104

Programs in basic medical sciences and clinical medicine for foreign medical graduates and students
Institution of Continuing Biomedical Education
222 E. Nineteenth St.
New York, NY 10003

Correspondence Services

FLEX Review Service
Box 24
Bronx, NY 10458

Medical Examination Publishing Company
65-36 Fresh Meadow Ln.
Flushing, NY 11365

Pre-test Service, Inc.
Box 330
Wallingford, CT 06492

Professional Examination Service
475 Riverside Dr.
New York, NY 10027

USNBE Review Center
Box 767
Friendswood, TX 77546

Appendix 36. Manufacturers of Audiovisual Educational Equipment

Bell and Howell
Audiovisual Products Division
7100 N. McCormack Rd.
Chicago, IL 60645
312-262-1600

Dukane Corp.
Audiovisual Division
2900 Dukane Dr.
St. Charles, IL 60174
312-584-2300

Eastman Kodak Co.
343 State St.
Rochester, NY 14560
716-325-2000

Milner-Fenwick, Inc.
2125 Greenspring Dr.
Timonium, MD 21093
800-638-8652

Singer Educational Systems
3750 Monroe Ave.
Rochester, NY 14630
716-586-2020

Appendix 37. Subscription Agency Services

EBSCO
Reception Room
Subscription Service
5350 Alpha Rd.
Dallas, TX 75250

F. W. Faxon Co., Inc.
15 Southwest Pk.
Westwood, MA 02090

Majors Scientific Books, Inc.
2221 Walnut Hill Ln.
P.O. Box 2700
Irving, TX 75061

Moore-Cottrell Subscription Agencies, Inc.
North Cohocton, NY 14868

Read-Moore Publication, Inc.
140 Cedar St.
New York, NY 10006

The purpose of this manual is to provide guidelines to familiarize all personnel with basic policies regarding employment in the practice. It is not intended to be an inflexible set of rules, but will serve as a guide to insure consistent and fair treatment of all employees. It will answer many questions you may have regarding job-related subjects. Please keep this manual for future reference.

Working Hours

The established working hours are from _____ to _____, Monday through Friday, with a designated lunch period of _____.

Full-time employees are expected to work forty hours per week; however, there may be times when an employee may be asked to work more than eight hours per day because of emergencies.

Personal Appearance and Cleanliness

An employee's personal appearance is an important part of public relations. Employee appearance and behavior will influence opinions held about this practice; each employee's daily appearance should reflect this consideration.

Cleanliness is also extremely important. Without special efforts the personnel in health care might actually contribute to the spread of disease. Good habits of hygiene not only reduce the possibility of disease transmission from one patient to another, but reduce the possibility of office personnel contracting illnesses from patients. The following guidelines are applicable to all employees:

1. *Hair.* Elaborate hair styles or ungroomed or dirty hair is not appropriate.
2. *Accessories.* Jewelry should be kept to a minimum. School, wedding and engagement rings, and wrist watches are appropriate. Small earrings, short necklaces, or simple pins may be worn.
3. *Fingernails.* The nails must be well cared for, clean, and neatly trimmed. Natural or clear polish is preferred. The nails should not be manicured at work.

Confidential Information

Information about patients, their illnesses, or their personal lives must be kept completely confidential. It is improper for an employee to reveal information about a patient, even to another member of the patient's family. If a patient asks questions about his or her case, refer the patient to the physician. Do not give advice to patients on personal matters—even when they ask for it.

When talking with a patient, manage the conversation in such a way that other patients who may be waiting will not overhear. Case histories, confidential papers, and even the appointment book should not be kept where passing patients may see them.

This office disapproves of gossip, whether personal or concerning a patient. Office matters should not be discussed outside of this office.

Personnel Confidentiality

Salaries, bonuses or raises, and performance evaluations are strictly confidential. This information is personal for each employee.

Personal Activities

The standards of efficiency are high for personnel in the medical field. There is seldom a moment when there is no work to be done. For this reason, employees are expected to postpone personal tasks until after work.

Occasionally, personal telephone calls may have to be received or made during business hours. A small number of such calls will be permitted, provided they are local and handled in such a manner as to not interfere with the employee's job responsibilities. Employees should keep such calls brief and be ready to interrupt them immediately to handle incoming calls and other business matters.

Probationary Period

Each new employee is on probation for the first ninety days of employment. Simply stated, this period provides the employee with an opportunity to see if he or she likes the work and can adjust to the environment. Similarly, this period provides the supervisor with an opportunity to see if the employee can adequately adapt to medical practice surroundings. A new employee having difficulty performing assigned duties should contact the physician/supervisor.

Termination

Any employee, probationary or permanent, committing a violation of one or more of the following rules will be dismissed without notice or severance pay.

1. Incompetence
2. Conviction of a major crime (felony)
3. Repeated or gross negligence in the performance of duty
4. Insubordination
5. Unjustified absenteeism
6. Embezzlement
7. Disorderly or unprofessional conduct
8. Working under the influence of alcohol
9. Falsification of information on his or her employment application
10. Destruction of office equipment
11. Falsification of time records
12. Misuse of controlled substances
13. Violation of confidential information

If an employee decides to terminate employment with the practice, the employee must submit a written resignation to the physician/supervisor at least ten working days prior to the resignation date. An employee who resigns with accumulated vacation time will be paid for this accumulated time.

Punctuality

Employees are expected to report promptly for work. Habitual tardiness by any employee will be cause for termination.

Employee Grievances

A channel for airing and seeking redress of employee grievances is provided by this office. If an employee has a grievance, he or she should contact the physician/supervisor, who will provide the employee with an opportunity to air the complaint in a private audience. The physician/supervisor will note all pertinent details, and after careful consideration, will make a decision with respect to the grievance.

Performance Reviews

Each employee's performance will be reviewed at twelve-month intervals. The physician/supervisor will schedule a time to interview each employee. This review will allow the supervisor and employee an opportunity to discuss the strengths and weaknesses of the employee's performance. Those areas of performance not up to standards will be monitored to insure improvement.

Salary Reviews

Salary reviews will be conducted for each employee annually. The salary review will be conducted by the physician/supervisor ninety days subsequent to the performance review. If economic conditions and the quality of the employee's work justify a salary adjustment, it will be given at this time. Such salary adjustments are made *for performance only.*

Civic Responsibilities

Whenever any employee is called for jury duty, the employee's full salary will continue during the period of jury duty, up to a maximum of two weeks. During this period, an amount will be deducted from the employee's salary to equal the total fees received from the government for jury services. If the jury duty continues beyond the two weeks, the practice will discontinue paying the employee's salary.

Employees wishing to vote on Election Day are expected to do so prior or subsequent to normal working hours.

Vacations: Full-Time Employees

Any employee who regularly works forty hours per week will be considered a full-time employee. Full-time employees are entitled to two weeks of vacation per year with pay, which accrues at the rate of ⅚ day of vacation per month of employment. If an employee leaves or is terminated during the first six months of employment, no vacation time will be accrued.

Vacations: Part-Time Employees

A part-time employee who works at least twenty hours per week will be entitled to two weeks of vacation pay, which accrues at the rate of 5/6 day per month of employment. If an employee leaves or is terminated during the first six months of employment, no vacation time will be accrued. A part-time employee will be paid an amount equal to the average weekly compensation paid during the six months preceding the vacation.

Miscellaneous Vacation Policies for All Employees

Requests for vacation should be made in writing to the physician/supervisor at least two weeks in advance of the desired vacation time. Every attempt will be made to accommodate an employee's request for vacation time.

If more than one employee requests a vacation for the same time period resulting in the office not being adequately staffed, the employee with seniority will be given first choice.

Accrued vacation will be computed based on the date of employment. An employee terminating employment after six months is entitled to receive vacation pay accrued to the date of termination unless the termination is the result of one or more reasons noted under the section entitled Termination.

An employee may be entitled to take one week of vacation time prior to its being accrued. If an employee subsequently terminates employment prior to accruing the week of vacation time, any vacation days taken but not accrued will be deducted from the employee's final paycheck.

Emergency Leave

Each request for emergency leave will be considered on its own merits. Leave normally will be granted with pay in the event of death or critical illness of spouse, children, or parents.

Leave may be granted without pay at the physician/supervisor's discretion for other purposes if application is made in writing, stating the reason and anticipated date of return.

Holidays

The office will normally be closed and full-time employees will be paid for each of these holidays: New Year's Day, Memorial Day, Independence Day, Labor Day, Thanksgiving Day, and Christmas Day. The employee must work the business day preceding and following the holiday, or have the physician/supervisor's approval of absence, in order to be paid for the holiday.

Sick Leave

An employee is eligible for sick leave with pay after three months of employment. Five days of sick leave with pay are granted each year. Sick leave is not cumulative and cannot be used as additional vacation time. Any sick leave will be recorded on the employee's attendance record. Sick leave that extends beyond the allowed amount will be regarded as time off without pay. At the end of the employment year, employees will be reimbursed for sick leave days not used.

Absences

When, for any reason, an employee cannot report for work, it is the employee's responsibility to telephone prior to working hours. Anyone absent for more than two consecutive days without contacting the supervisor will no longer be considered an employee of this practice.

Employees are expected to handle personal matters such as doctor's visits on their days off. There may be special occasions, however, when an employee needs a few hours off during the workday to attend to personal matters. Such a request should be made of the physician/supervisor; and, if permission is given, the following will apply:

1. The employee may elect to use this time as vacation, in the case of a full day off.
2. The employee may elect to make the lost time up—within thirty days of the date the time off was taken.
3. The employee may elect to take this time off without pay.

Medical Care

Minor illnesses of employees will be treated in the office without charge. Any laboratory work that can be handled in the office will also be done without charge. Employees are encouraged to seek medical advice and treatment quite early in the onset of an illness or suspected illness, to avoid the development of more serious problems.

Each employee should have a personal physician other than a physician in the office in order that complete and objective treatment can be given without interfering with the employer-employee relationship. If an employee has no personal physician the doctor will suggest one.

Maternity Leave

Employees who become pregnant may work up until the time they deliver. The employee will be granted a six-week leave of absence. Although continued employment cannot be guaranteed when the employee wishes to return to work, every effort will be made by the supervisor/physician to rehire the employee. The supervisor/physician can provide information about maternity and disability benefits available to the employee during her leave of absence. When an employee takes a leave of absence for reasons of pregnancy the employee will receive any accrued sick leave and vacation time pay.

Insurance Coverage

After a ninety-day probationary period, each employee will be enrolled in the office health care plan. This plan provides health insurance coverage and a life insurance policy at no cost to the employee.

Pay Periods

All employees will be paid biweekly for regular time worked. Remuneration for authorized overtime will be paid by special check at the end of the month. When the pay period ends on a holiday, employees will be paid on the previous day. Deductions will be withheld for income tax and Social Security.

Retirement Plans

This practice has established a retirement plan for the benefit of all full-time employees who have worked for a period of _____ consecutive months. The contributions to the retirement plan are made by the employer, except those contributions that you are permitted to make on a voluntary basis. Voluntary contributions are not required and will not affect the contributions made by the employer.

All monies paid into the plan are administered by the trustee of the plan. Each year that you are a member of the retirement plan, you acquire a _____ percent interest in the funds set aside for your benefit. After _____ years of participation, you will be entitled to all of the benefits in your account. When you reach age 65, die, or become permanently disabled, you or your beneficiary will receive 100 percent of your account. Each year you will receive a written statement of your account for your share of the plan. If you have any questions about this statement of account, please contact the physician/supervisor or the trustee of the plan. Copies of the retirement plan are available if you wish to consult your employer or tax advisor regarding the effect of this plan on your overall tax situation.

This information has been prepared to inform an employee of benefits and privileges as well as standards and procedures of this office. The provisions of this office policy manual apply equally to all employees.

We welcome any questions you may have and hope that you will enjoy your employment with us.

Index